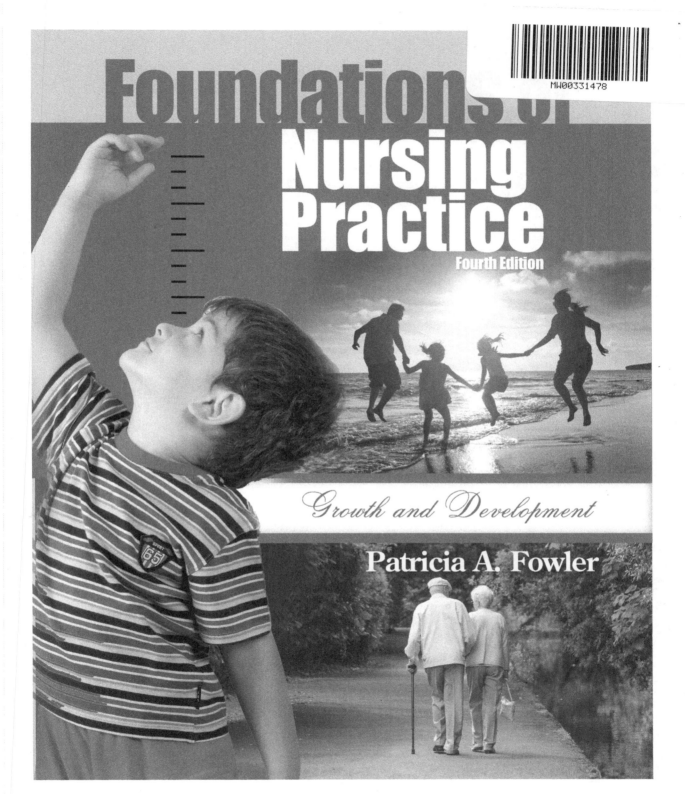

Foundations of

Nursing
Practice

Fourth Edition

Growth and Development

Patricia A. Fowler

Kendall Hunt
publishing company

Cover image © Shutterstock, Inc.

Kendall Hunt
publishing company

www.kendallhunt.com
Send all inquiries to:
4050 Westmark Drive
Dubuque, IA 52004-1840

Copyright © 2011, 2012, 2016, 2018 by Kendall Hunt Publishing Company

ISBN 978-1-5249-5973-9

Published in the United States of America

Contents

Introduction

Health, by definition of the World Health Organization (WHO), is the bio-psycho-social, cultural, and spiritual well-being of man, and not just the absence of disease. Individuals with physiologic health but lacking in psycho-social health are not really healthy. Individuals who are psychologically well, but have multiple physiologic problems, are not healthy either.

Nursing is a profession that is committed to health from a holistic perspective. This means that nurses are called upon to address the needs of the whole person. In order to do this, nurses need to know psychology, philosophy, sociology, religion, and culture, as well as the sciences of anatomy, physiology, and chemistry.

Knowledge of Growth and Development is essential to addressing the holistic health needs of individuals across the lifespan. The human body undergoes multiple changes throughout life. With each change, there is the resultant demand for physiological and/or psychological adaptation. Some changes improve body strength and stability and resistance, while others actually detract from or limit these assets. With each physiologic change, there is a demand for adaptation and/or change in cognitive and psychosocial perspective, that is, how well the individual accepts the change. Similarly, psychological issues impact on the physiological health of the body. Change in any human dimension simply does not exist without impacting all of the other dimensions.

Growth and Development integrates the anatomical and physiologic changes that occur at different stages of life with the psycho-social-cultural demands that accompany these changes. Growth and Development knowledge helps the nurse to recognize the very wide ranges of normal. With this insight, nurses can anticipate expected responses. Growth and Development knowledge also helps nurses to gain insight into the apparent signs (symptoms and behaviors) that are indicative of actual or potential problems so they can intervene in a timely, effective manner.

Nursing interventions to promote health, prevent disease, restore and/or maintain health, are only effective if they are founded on accurate assessments. Growth and Development knowledge is an essential component of a comprehensive, holistic assessment. Growth and Development knowledge facilitates nurses in their goal of meeting the unique, holistic needs of individuals across the life span.

In the following pages, Growth and Development will be discussed from a nursing perspective, that is, from the perspective of what nurses need to know in order to accurately assess and appropriately respond to individual needs across the life span. This discussion is not intended to cover everything there is to know about Growth and Development. This discussion is not all inclusive or exclusive—it is simply a condensed version of what I have found to be helpful in my nursing career.

Patricia Fowler, MSN, RN

Growth and Development Overview

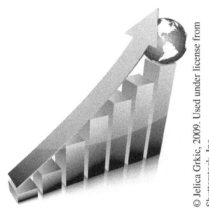

© Jelica Grkic, 2009. Used under license from Shutterstock, Inc.

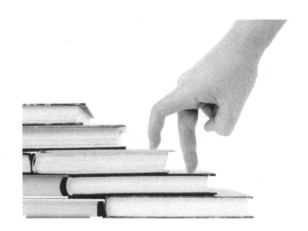

© Tatiana Popova, 2009. Used under license from Shutterstock, Inc.

Objectives

Upon completion of this chapter, the reader should be able to:

1. Describe factors contributing to progression in Growth and Development theory.
2. Define common terms associated with Growth and Development theory.
3. Describe the value of Growth and Development theory in nursing assessment for patients across the life span.
4. Explain the interrelationship between the theories of Erikson, Piaget, and Kohlberg as related to Growth and Development theory.
5. Identify and describe the major stages (crises) of Erikson's psychosocial theory.
6. Identify and explain the major stages of Piaget's theory of cognition.
7. Identify and explain the major stages of Kohlberg's theory of morality.

Key Terms

Asynchronous growth: not all parts of our body grow at the same rate and time

Cephalocaudal: growth proceeding from head to tail

Development: an increase in complexity and/or maturation of behavior

Exposure: the genetic predispositions that either increase or decrease our reaction to stressors in the environment

General-to-Specific Development: the manner of progression in refinement of movement, for example, babies respond with both arms and legs, then progress to just arms, then to one arm, one hand, and ultimately to a pincer grasp (thumb-finger precision).

Growth: the increase in size or number of cells, organs, bodies

Nature: the Growth and Development forces that are genetically inherited

Nurture: the Growth and Development forces that evolve with environmental exposure

Progressive differentiation and autonomy: a description of human progression that is characterized by an increased uniqueness related to the extent of our interaction with one another.

Proximodistal: growth proceeding near to far meaning that it proceeds from the midline to the lateral extremities

Sequential growth: progressive and sequential increase in size meaning that growth cannot be reversed or un-done

Simple-to-Complex Development: the manner of progression in complexity of movement, for example, we stand before we walk and we walk before we run. In language, we proceed from one word to two, to simple phrases, to simple sentences, to compound sentences.

Susceptibility: the environmental influences that either increase or decrease our genetic potential

Symmetrical growth: appearance that is balanced and aligned proportionately to a central axis

---

Growth and Development Theory Related to Optimal Nursing Care

Nursing is very different from medicine. Nurses facilitate the patient's response to a disease or condition rather than just treat the disease or condition, that is, nurses treat the whole person. Since individuals respond to wellness or illness uniquely, a holistic approach to patient care necessitates consideration of the unique bio-psycho-cultural-social-religious aspects involved. Because this holistic approach is applicable to everyone across the life span, nurses must also have a solid understanding of Growth and Development theory.

Growth and Development is evidenced in *behavior*. So nurses need to have a good understanding of the principles of Growth and Development in order to respond to each individual's response pattern. Without assessing the developmental stages of the individual, nurses cannot individualize care.

Human behavior is unique to each individual but we all have some shared basic needs. Maslow (1968) has **prioritized** these needs as Survival (food, water, air), Safety (protection from environmental risks), Security (feeling of stability and being loved), Self-esteem (pride in accomplishments), and Self-actualization (reaching our greatest potential).

Shared human behavior is also characterized by being **directional** (purposeful and striving for potential). Everything that we do is for a reason as opposed to behavior that is reflexive or by instinct. Human behavior is also irreversible. We can always say that we are sorry, but it never takes away the action itself. We can never undo anything that we do.

Some human behavior may be shared only in some locales. For example, depending on where you live, the standards may be different. Because behavior is reflective of cultural and societal norms, some behaviors are judged according to the "rules" of the day. For example, smoking used to be a sign that you were with the times, but now in the United States, it is considered essentially taboo. In France, smoking is still very well tolerated. Pregnant adolescents in the United States used to be hidden away, but now they are welcomed into their regular high school classes. Homosexual, lesbian and transgender behaviors were once deemed aberrant but are now commonly accepted as is same sex marriage.

The greatest principle of human behavior is that it is reflective of **progressive differentiation and autonomy**. This means that, because of our expanding human interactions, the more we become unique. We need to understand others in order to understand ourselves and we also need to understand ourselves in order to understand others. This dichotomy is very evident in personal perception and in the way we communicate and react to others.

Growth vs. Development

So are Growth and Development one and the same? What are the differences between *growth* and *development*? Why are the terms *growth* and *development* usually grouped together?

Growth and Development are VERY different, but generally speaking, are very interdependent. When growth occurs, it is often and usually accompanied by developmental maturation as well. So growth may precede developmental maturation or it may be in reverse and/or growth and development can be simultaneous.

Growth has a strong genetic (nature) component especially when speaking physiologically. Organ development and innate vulnerability or immunity to disease have definite familial links. On the other hand, the development of many psycho-social and cognitive traits (also genetic) are highly influenced by external forces (nurture).

The influencing factors of Growth and Development have been studied extensively throughout the years. Some argue that nature (genetics) has the greatest influence and others claim that it is nurture (environmental stimuli) that dictates how and when we grow and develop.

Nature vs. Nurture

So is Growth and Development more influenced by **nature** or **nurture**? Growth is largely influenced by genetics (nature). If our parents are tall, we most likely will be tall. If our parents are small boned, it is likely that we will be too. Nutrition is also a major factor in growth. Without protein, fat, carbohydrates, vitamins, and minerals, the body will not grow. But this is nurture. Sleep is also a major factor in growth. The nissel substance produced during sleep is required for both linear and cellular growth (this is nature) but establishing restful sleep patterns is nurture. Failure to thrive, or failure to grow, is also closely linked to nurturing, bonding, and affection. This is often seen in newborns who do not seem to connect with their primary caregivers. This is also seen in older depressed individuals who perceive themselves as being unloved.

What do you think?

A 24-year-old woman who had a strong family history of type 2 diabetes (virtually every female in three generations developed this disease by age 35) consciously chose to control her weight through healthy dietary choices and an exercise regimen. At age 46, she still did not have diabetes. Is this nurture overcoming nature?

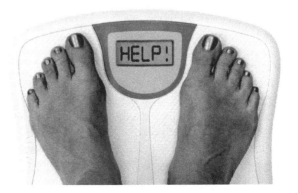

© Amy Walters, 2009. Used under license from Shutterstock, Inc.

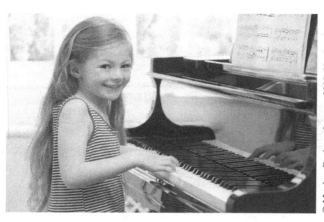

© Monkey Business Images, 2009. Used under license from Shutterstock, Inc.

There is no clear delineation of impact of nature and/or nurture. Nature and nurture, in reality, are totally interdependent on one another. Growth and Development require a combination of physical, cognitive, emotional, and socio-cultural factors. Within this framework, it is apparent that two major issues emerge: susceptibility and exposure.

Susceptibility refers to the environmental influences that either increase or decrease our genetic potential. For example, even though I may have a genetic predisposition to diabetes, I can decrease that potential by choosing optimal nutrition and by exercising. Another example might be that I have a genetic tendency to be a great musician but if I never get the opportunity to learn how to play an instrument, then this potential is lost.

Exposure, on the other hand, refers to the genetic predispositions that either increase or decrease our reaction to stressors in the environment. For example, I may not have a genetic predisposition to diabetes, but because of poor nutrition and sedentary lifestyle, I could increase this risk potential. Another example would be vaccines. My genetic predisposition would leave me vulnerable to some very serious communicable diseases, but by being exposed to immunizations, I have now decreased that risk potential.

Genetics, as explained by the Mendellian law of dominant and recessive genes, (Bateson, W. 1901) dictates the color of our skin, what color eyes we have, how tall we will be, and whether or not our hair is straight or curly. Genetics, with its heterozygous and homozygous genes, can also dictate some immunity factors, such as predisposition to certain diseases.

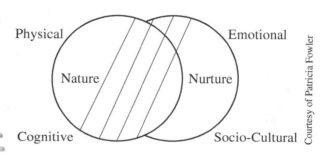

Physical — Emotional

Nature   Nurture

Cognitive — Socio-Cultural

Courtesy of Patricia Fowler

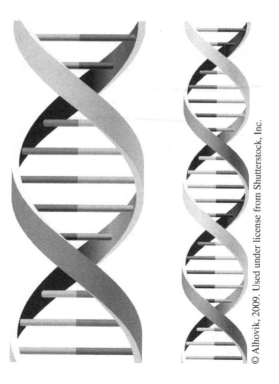

© Alhovik, 2009. Used under license from Shutterstock, Inc.

Genetics also plays a role in our cognitive ability related to the configuration of our brain cells. Similarly, the hormones that are genetically based regulate our biorhythms and can be seen to influence our emotional and personality tendencies.

Nurture (environmental stimuli), on the other hand, contributes to how we use what we have inherited genetically. The geographical location in which we live, the educational level, and economic ability of our parents that allows them to provide adequate nutrition and the amount of exposure to multiple experiences in life, the degree of parenting skills used in our upbringing, and societal norms all definitely contribute to who we are today.

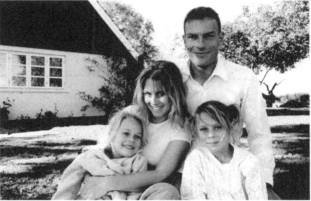

So let's define the terms *growth* and *development*. **Growth** is an increase in size or number. We usually think about growth only in terms of height, but it applies to other increases as well. (Body Organs, Parts) For example, cells multiply to form more cells, which can also become larger cells. Even with body dysfunction such as with cancer, the tumor cells are growing inside us. The brain grows substantially in size to accommodate the increased number of neurons and amount of cerebral spinal fluid required to make us functional. That is why infants have the "soft spots" on their heads—the skull has not yet closed because the brain is still growing. The stomach grows larger to allow a greater intake of nutrients that allows us to eat at less frequent

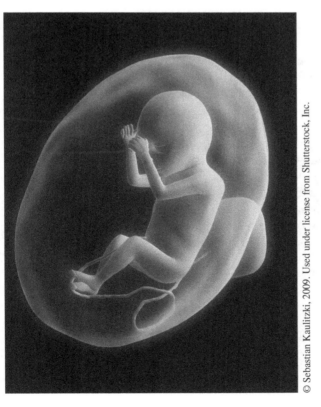

intervals. The lungs grow larger to allow a greater intake of oxygen that is required for greater energy and endurance. The heart grows larger to produce a greater circulatory output to reach the rest of our growing body, and muscles and fat increase to help us grow in weight. All of this occurs as well as the legs becoming longer to increase our height. Growth means greater size or greater number.

So what do we need to know about Growth? Growth is **cephalocaudal** (head to tail) meaning that it proceeds from the head down. This is very apparent when one considers fetal growth in utero. The head is the first discernible body part and remains extremely large in comparison to the rest of the developing body. It is only after the head is formed that the trunk becomes apparent and then the growth of the arms, and then the growth of the legs.

Growth is also **proximodistal** (near to far), meaning that it proceeds from the midline to the extremities. This is also apparent in utero when the growth of the head and trunk precede the growth of arms and legs. This is a term used commonly in describing the direction of movement of an individual.

Body growth is also **symmetrical** in that our appearance is balanced. For example, our ribs are aligned proportionately on the right side and on the left side, our arms and legs are the same length, and our shoulders are straight across. When there are anatomical deviations from this symmetrical appearance, it usually requires "fixing" through braces, surgery, or use of assistive devices such as crutches, wheel chairs, or canes.

Growth is **sequential**. This simply means that growth cannot be undone. Once we have arms and legs, they do not un-grow. Growth may become stunted but it does not undo. It is a fact that some height may be lost during the elder years, but this is related to a decrease in the fluid cushioning in the vertebrae of the spine. This decrease causes the vertebrae to settle in closer to one another and results in a decrease in height.

Growth is also **asynchronous**. This means that not all parts of our body grow at the same rate and time. In fact, different parts of our bodies grow faster than other parts at different times of our lives. For example, preteens usually demonstrate a dramatic growth in shoe (foot) size before it is apparent that there is growth in the long leg bones. It is amazing how nature prepares the body for what is about to occur. We definitely need bigger feet to support our bigger bodies! We also see a less dramatic version of a height spurt in preschoolers, especially as compared to the relatively slow height increase during the toddler years. And as you know, once the epiphysis closes on the long bones, our height has reached its maximum level.

> *Did you know?*
>
> It is during Infancy and Puberty that there is faster growth and more diverse change in the body than in any other age frame.

Development, on the other hand, refers to an increase in complexity and/or maturation. For example, the neurons in the brain progressively connect to allow us to process information in a more complex manner. Our muscles progressively develop to increase our strength, endurance, flexibility, and coordination. Our organs progressively develop to higher levels of functioning, such as the kidneys developing increased concentration and filtration, the stomach progressively developing by producing the enzymes necessary to facilitate digestion, and the endocrine system developing an extremely complex feedback mechanism for regulation of all the body's hormones.

Development proceeds in a **general-to-specific** manner. This is evident in simple movement. Initially babies respond with both arms and legs, then progress to just arms, then to one arm, one hand, and ultimately to a pincer grasp (thumb-finger precision). This is also evident in the fact that the large muscles develop before the small muscles and so gross motor skills like walking, running, and climbing precede the fine motor skills of holding a crayon and forming defined letters.

Development also follows a **simple-to-complex** format. For example, we stand before we walk and we walk before we run. In language, we proceed from one word to two, to simple phrases, to simple sentences, to compound sentences. In math, we proceed from simple addition to subtraction, then to multiplication and division, then to fractions, algebra, geometry, and calculus.

As nurses, we can contribute to growth by monitoring, implementing, and teaching about optimal nutrition and rest. Equally important is the monitoring and teaching about nurture. Essential to nurture is exposure, opportunity, stimulation, and guidance; these are best described in the developmental theories. Understanding what psychological, cognitive, and moral perspectives usually exist in individuals at certain ages or at different stages in their developmental progress helps the nurse to better help patients during health and disease.

Developmental Theorists

The psychosocial theory of Erik Erikson (1968), the cognitive theory of Jean Piaget (1950), and the moral theory of Kohlberg (1969) have been found to be valid criteria for assisting nurses in making these assessments and in facilitating patient response.

Erik Erikson: Psychosocial Theory

Erik Erikson was a student of Sigmund Freud. Even though the psycho-sexual theory of Freud is alluded to minimally in today's health care, it was and is a strong influence on Erikson's perspective. For example, when Freud referred to the Oral Stage (Infancy), he indicated that infants needed to experience gratification through their mouth (sucking and eating) and that if they didn't receive full gratification, that this could result in oral fixations later in life such as with overeating and/or alcoholism. Erikson, on the other hand, states that infants need to receive food and drink from their primary caregivers in order to establish a sense of trust.

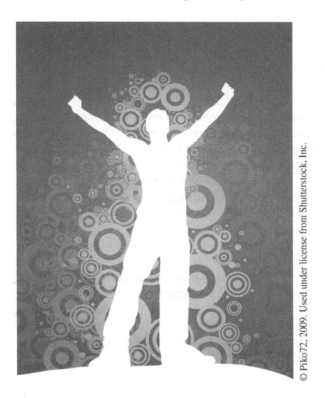

© Piko72, 2009. Used under license from Shutterstock, Inc.

Freud's Anal Stage (toddler), focuses on holding on and letting go and is highly connected with the rigidity of toilet training. If not properly accomplished, this could result in adults being very opinionated, stingy and self centered. On the other hand, Erikson states that to achieve autonomy, the toddler needs to gain control of his body, his emotions, and his sphincters. Similarly while Freud referred to the Oedipal Stage (preschool), as having some fixation on parents of the opposite sex, Erikson simply states that, in striving for initiative, that preschoolers often imitate the same-sexed parent to compete for the affection of the opposite sexed parent. This is the Oedipal complex.

So Freud's theory persists in many ways through Erikson's psychosocial theory. Erikson just de-emphasizes the sexual aspects. Freud indicated that many adult "mental" issues were related to a fixation at one of the early stages of development; that is, oral personalities evolved because there were unmet needs during the infancy "sucking" stage or that anal personalities evolved because there was too much emphasis on toilet training during toddlerhood. Erikson, similarly, states that it is essential for individuals to resolve the crisis of each stage before progressing successfully to the next. For example, Erikson theorizes that, unless an infant accomplishes trust, they cannot progress to becoming autonomous (the task of the toddler). Erikson identifies each stage as a crisis that must be dealt with and so identifies outcomes as either positive or negative. (See Developmental Theorists chart at the end of this chapter).

Jean Piaget: Theory of Cognition

Jean Piaget (1950) is credited with the development of a theory of cognition. This theory attempts to explain how we take in information, assimilate the new data with what we have previously learned and experienced, and accommodate the new information for application to new situations. The principal stages of Piaget's theory are Reflexive, Sensorimotor, Preoperational, Concrete Operations, and Formal Operations.

In the **Reflexive Stage**, there are spontaneous neuromuscular movements but no purposeful movements. Mouths suck, eyes blink, arms and legs jerk in response to loud noises, arms and legs retract when painful stimuli are introduced, and fingers grasp. The sucking, moro, rooting, grasping and dancing reflexes are discussed in greater detail in the Chapter on Infancy.

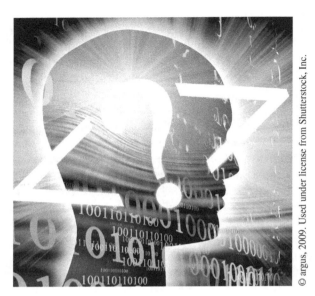

© argus, 2009. Used under license from Shutterstock, Inc.

In the **Sensorimotor Stage**, infants and toddlers use their senses (touch, taste, smell, sight, and hearing) to learn. For example, an infant would examine a new object visually, pick it up to see how it feels, smell it for any distinguishing odor, shake it to see if it makes any sound, and then probably put it in their mouth to see what it tastes like. They then compare it to other objects that they have previously explored and realign their thought processes to see where it fits. Information is then organized into the brain's memory cells in a classification system. The sensorimotor stage has five sub-stages: Primary Circular reaction, Secondary Circular reaction, Coordination of secondary schemata, Tertiary Circular reaction and Solutions via mental combinations.

In the Primary Circular sub-stage, an infant may experience a unique sound or texture or action totally by accident. For example, they may touch a bell on the mobile above their crib and hear the tinkling sound and they like it. Or with regard to texture, they might discover the softness of a stuffed animal or the rigidity of a rattle. It is the discovery of this new experience that makes them want to replicate the experience. So they may purposefully touch the bell on the mobile again. They purposely reach for the stuffed toy or rattle again. This is secondary circular reaction. When they have been successful in creating this sensation, they then store this in their memory so they can repeat this pleasurable sensation at will. This is called Coordination of secondary schemata. That is, they have put two and two together to remember that a particular action results in something pleasurable.

The Coordination of secondary schemata may not be so pleasurable when parents attempt to hide a toy or bottle from an infant, and the infant remembers where it was. There is also a negative response when parents leave the infant in the care of someone else. The infant remembers where Mom or Dad are supposed to be and when they are not there, this can be quite traumatic. Tertiary circular reaction and Solutions via mental combinations are expansions of this memory to beginning problem solving. Coordination of secondary schemata and solutions via mental combinations could also become safety issues if the infant needs to climb to retrieve objects that they want.

In the Preoperational Stage, problem solving relies less on physical manipulation of objects and there is increased use of memory, language, and intuition. For example, a preschooler would examine an object and classify it according to their memory of similar objects. There is still some trial-and-error experimentation but this level of cognition allows young children to anticipate and figure out some possibilities without physical manipulation.

Centering is one of the limitations in the Preoperational Stage of thinking. Centering means that individuals can usually only focus on one aspect of a situation at a time. For example, when learning what it means that someone is their brother, they cannot simultaneously understand that this same individual may be someone else's son or nephew. Preoperational thinking would also preclude individuals from defining an object from multiple perspectives. For example, a ball is something that is round or something that can bounce, but most children in this stage would not identify both aspects.

In the Concrete Operations Stage, school-age children use their memory and newly acquired skills to demonstrate skill. It is in this stage that children like to manipulate numbers (as in learning the basic skills of mathematics), dates (as in learning basic time lines of history), and classification (as in filing concepts to organizational subsets). School-age children also love to manipulate letters to form new words making hand-writing and spelling attractive subjects. Locating countries and continents on globes or maps is also a hands-on skill that links memory with identification.

Some of the characteristic capabilities of Concrete Operations include reversibility and conservation of matter. The concept of **reversibility** means that school-age children can understand that subtraction is the reverse of addition and that division is the reverse of multiplication, that is, actions can be reversed.

Conservation of matter refers to understanding that some things can change form but still remain the same. For example, water can be frozen but still remain water and clay can be shaped into forms but it is still clay. Another example is that the same amount of water in two different sized containers is still the same amount of water. Undoubtedly, a preschooler would claim that the amount of water in a tall, slender glass was greater than the amount of water in a short glass with a greater diameter, even when they are shown that the amounts of water were equal before being transferred into these containers.

School-age children are also capable of **sorting and ranking** objects according to color, size, importance, and/or value. For example, a school-age child could sort coins according to size, recognizing that the dime is the smallest and the half-dollar as the largest. When sorting according to value, the penny is identified as the least. A preschooler would undoubtedly prefer to have ten pennies rather than one dime because, in their thinking, more is better.

In the Formal Operations Stage, adolescents begin to think about thinking. They are now capable of hypothesizing about possibilities. This is why they can now make choices based on an assessment of the anticipated outcomes. They can choose the academic courses they need to take to prepare themselves for college or select a college to apply to, based on the curriculum, opportunities, and/or their career goals. They can choose extracurricular activities based on their own personal interests or talents and choose part-time job work settings that fit their schedules and provide them with extra money for personal wants.

They also understand that activities have consequences. This is why most adolescents sometimes choose to break rules understanding that they live with the repercussions. Breaking curfew and being grounded could very readily appear "worth" it when they are having an unusually good time. On the other hand, most adolescents have a sense of "immunity" to less than desirable consequences. For example, many adolescents experiment with sexual activity without using protection because they truly believe that they are being careful or that pregnancy and/or sexually transmitted disease surely would not happen to them. Adolescents may also ignore speed limits because they assume they have superior control of their vehicles or experiment with alcohol because they think they can hold their own.

Because the brain reaches maximum growth and development by puberty, cognition also reaches a peak capacity. This is called **fluid intelligence**. Problem solving skills improve and wiser choices are more evident with increased age and experience throughout the young adult, middle adult and elder years, so even though the formal operations stage of cognition remains constant, there emerges a **crystallized intelligence** (wisdom). (See Developmental Theorists chart at the end of this chapter).

Formal Operations is the final stage of Piaget's theory of cognition but it is not complete during the adolescent stage. With age and experience comes wisdom and discrimination. So young adults, middle-aged adults, and elders continue to expand the possibilities of alternative choices and consequences and continue to become skilled in organizing details of strategies and become more structured and disciplined in embarking on these choices.

Lawrence Kohlberg: Theory on Morality

Lawrence Kohlberg's (1969) theory of morality is based somewhat on Piaget's theory of cognition and was based on an extensive study of young boys. Gilligan (1982) similarly studied girls and found Kohlberg's theory generally applicable but in some stages, devoid of a caring perspective, that is more commonly associated with the female gender.

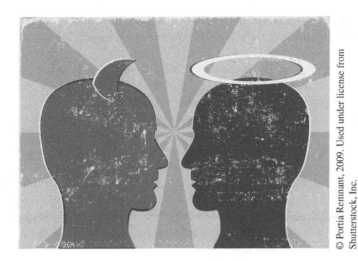

© Portia Remnant, 2009. Used under license from Shutterstock, Inc.

Kohlberg and Gilligan agree that the level of morality that can be achieved by any individual is dependent upon the individual's ability to process information. For example, young children (under the age of 3), because of their egotistical frame of reference, cannot understand that something is nice or not nice. They only see actions from their perspective.understanding another's perspective.

That is why young children, who do not understand 'cause and effect", simply cannot understand the meaning of danger and must be protected through supervision and the provision of safe play environments. They also cannot understand "sharing" of their toys. Likewise, individuals who are incapable of understanding societal norms cannot be accountable for some of their choices. For example, for someone with limited cognitive ability, picking their nose in public would not be perceived as unacceptable behavior.

Kohlberg's morality, like Piaget's theory, has stages that are progressive in that, the greater one's ability to process information, the higher level of morality that can be achieved. But, in opposition to Erikson and Piaget, Kohlberg clearly states that even though individuals are capable of higher levels of morality, they do not always behave at that stage. They very often return to very basic levels of morality, especially when pressured.

It is important to note that Kohlberg's theory on morality relates to an individual's perspective and potential ability to assume responsibility for their actions, but does not address the many factors that often influence one's personal perspective of morality. These include societal norms, family and child rearing values and religious upbringing.

Societal norms are different in countries around the world and some have evolved over time resulting in altered social expectations. Examples of changing societal norms include acceptance or disapproval of smoking or drinking, nudity, cursing and violence in public and in films. Societal norms also address acceptance or disallowance of sexual harassment when and wherever, acceptance or disallowance of bigotry to the LGBTQ community or of any minority group (based on color, race or religion), and acceptance or disallowance of same sex unions/marriages.

Examples of family and child rearing values include emphasis on sharing, honesty and integrity versus lying, stealing and greed. Religious upbringing relates to a formation of a correct conscience based on biblical guidelines.

Kohlberg's first stage of morality is simply "amoral," meaning that morality is not even factored into the picture. This is the stage normally assigned to infants who perform actions from the perspective of "if it feels good, do it." So if I am hungry, I cry. If I don't like my food, I throw it on the floor. If I am doing something I like and you interrupt me, then I am unhappy and then I scream and cry or throw a temper tantrum. Many adults sometimes act at this stage when they selfishly put their own desires above the wants and needs of others.

It is often stated that an infant cannot be spoiled. But by the time young children emerge into toddlerhood, it is important for them to learn the difference between what is acceptable and what is not. Teaching morality to young children is not an easy task but an essential task to facilitate socialization and healthy choices. Parents need to be constantly reminded to show the child that it is the action that is not acceptable but that the child is **always** loved.

The next stage is known as Preconventional and is divided into two levels: "punishment and obedience" and "instrumental purpose and exchange." In the punishment and obedience stage, typically ascribed to toddlers and young children, individuals behave only to avoid the consequences of punishment. Children, not quite convinced that they shouldn't do whatever they feel like doing as in the previous stage, now do what they can get away with. They are "good" only as long as someone is watching but do what they want when that pressure is not apparent. As long as no one is seeing what they are doing, it is okay to do what they want. For example, a child may not openly hit a younger sibling when the parents are watching because they know that they will be rebuked with a verbal "no" or a scornful look or "time-out." But when the parents are not around, it is not uncommon for them to hit or bite or inflict some type of injury.

It is not only young children who act in this realm. Have you ever exceeded the speed limit just because you knew there were no police around? Or have you turned in an assignment just because you didn't want to fail a course? This, too, is morality at the stage of punishment and obedience.

The other Preconventional Stage, according to Kohlberg, is "instrumental purpose and exchange." In this stage, preschoolers perform "good" acts to receive praise from their parents or teachers. Children learn to impress others with their behavior. That is why preschoolers love to show off by performing acrobatics or telling stories or helping Mommy and Daddy around the house. They want to hear how "good" they are or they want to earn a reward. Very often, parents forget that children thrive for the praise associated with these actions and that they don't necessarily need a trip to McDonald's or a piece of candy or money to put in their piggy banks. If children become too accustomed to receiving rewards for every good deed, it may be very difficult to get them to do anything around the house unless there is a reward involved.

Similarly, most of us are guilty of performing good actions because we want others to see how "good" we are or how efficient we are or how valuable we are. This is important to our self-esteem but is also evident of a very limited morality. It is also at this stage when young children very often confuse intention and accident. For example, spilling a glass of milk when reaching for it does not make them a bad person, but because of the reaction of others (yelling or screaming), young children cannot differentiate. It is extremely important for parents to remember that accidents do happen.

School-age children are obsessed with rules. They become very upset when rules (even board game rules) are broken. Rules are made to be observed and there is no excuse for any alternative. School-age children are notorious for tattling on others because they did not follow the rules. This emphasizes the "good girl, bad boy" frame of reference.

This is the Conventional Stage of morality in which the Golden Rule "do unto others as you would have them do unto you" dominates. Lying sometimes comes into the picture during this stage because it is unacceptable to be labeled as "bad," so individuals lie about what they did or didn't do. There are, unfortunately, many adults who function at this level of morality without giving any credit to the circumstances that may have led up to the action. For example, is it equally bad for someone to steal a loaf of bread when one individual thought it was a lark while another was truly hungry? This is the stage in which Gilligan found the gender difference most apparent. She claims that females are generally more understanding of the caring modality.

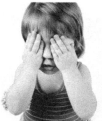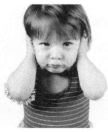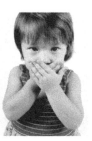

© Liudmila P. Sundikova, 2009. Used under license from Shutterstock, Inc.

The Postconventional Stage of Kohlberg's morality is described as "doing the right thing for the right reason." This simply means that as we expand our experience and knowledge; that is, because of achieving formal operations, we are capable of understanding what is humanly right. So we are capable of treating all other humans with total respect and dignity without discrimination or bias. Yet exclusion, discrimination, and deprivation routinely occur in our society. So even though morality is progressive in sync with our cognition, there is absolutely no direct indication that we are acting at these levels. (See Developmental Theorists chart at the end of this chapter).

Summary

Growth and Development theory is essential to optimal Nursing care because it explains so much about human behavior and responses. This helps the nurse to better individualize care. There are many theories on growth and development but the three addressed in this chapter (Erikson's Psychosocial theory, Piaget's Theory on Cognition and Kohlberg's Theory on Morality) are the most established and credible theories known and used in health care delivery practice.

Comparison and Parallels of Developmental Theorists

The following chart parallels the theories of Erikson, Piaget, and Kohlberg. Generally speaking, there is identified an approximate age that is associated with each of the theorists' stages. Yet this shows potential more so than actuality, especially related to morality where actions fluctuate relative to the self-esteems of the individual as well as to their level of cognition (indicated by the reciprocal arrows).

Developmental Theorists

Stage	*Erikson*	*Piaget*	*Kohlberg*
Infancy 0–1 month 1–4 months 4–8 months 8–12 months 12–15 months	**Trust vs. Mistrust**	**Reflexive Sensorimotor** 1. Primary circular reaction 2. Secondary circular reaction 3. Coordination of secondary schemata (object permanence) 4. Tertiary circular reaction	**Amoral**
Toddler **(15 months–3 years)** (15–24 months) (24–36 months)	**Autonomy vs. Shame & Doubt**	5. Solutions via mental combinations	**Preconventional** 1. Punishment vs. Obedience
Preschool **(3–5 years)**	**Initiative vs. Guilt**	**Preoperational** a. Preconceptual (representational thought/language) b. Intuitive (use of symbolism)	2. Instrumental Purpose & Exchange
School Age **(6–12 years)**	**Industry vs. Inferiority**	**Concrete Operations** (ordering, classifying, reversibility, conservation)	**Conventional** 3. Conformity Golden Rule
Adolescent **(11–18 years)**	**Identity vs. Role Diffusion**	**Formal Operations** (capability of abstract thought & futuristic plans but inexperience limits implementation)	4. Social System & Development of Conscience
Young Adult **(18–35 years)**	**Intimacy vs. Isolation**	(now capable of formulating realistic plans and means to accomplish them)	**Postconventional** 5. Social Contract & Utility
Middle-Age Adult **(35–65 years)**	**Generativity vs. Stagnation**	*Fluid Intelligence vs. Crystallized Intelligence*	6. Universal Ethical Principles ??
Elderly **(65+ years)**	**Integrity vs. Despair**	*Fluid Intelligence vs. Crystallized Intelligence*	

References

Bateson, William (1901) Translation of Mendel, Gregor. 1866. Versuche über Plflanzenhybriden. Verhandlungen des naturforschenden Vereines in Brünn, Bd. IV für das Jahr 1865, Abhandlungen, 3–47.

Erikson, E. H. (1968). *Childhood and society* (35th anniversary ed.). New York: Norton.

Gilligan, C. (1982). *In a different voice: Psychological theory and women's development*. Cambridge, MA: Harvard University Press.

Kohlberg, L. (1981). *The philosophy of moral development: Vol. 1*. San Francisco: Harper & Row.

Maslow, A. (1968). *Toward a psychology of being* (2nd ed.). New York: Van Nostrand-Reinhold.

Piaget, J. (1950). *The psychology of intelligence*. London: Routledge and Kegan Paul.

Reflection

In the space below, think about yourself and describe how or why you think you have turned out the way you are. Was it mostly nature or nurture?

Assignment

Search to find Carol Gilligan's theory of morality and write a brief comparison of her theory with that of Lawrence Kohlberg.

Name: _____

Study Guide for Growth and Development Overview

1. Define 'GROWTH' and give one example of how/when growth occurs in the human body.

2. Define 'DEVELOPMENT' and give one example of how/when development occurs in human ability/ capability.

3. Explain why E. Erikson calls each of his stages 'CRISES'.

4. Explain simple to complex development and give at least one example.

5. Explain cephalocaudal growth and give at least one example.

6. Define progressive differentiation and explain how it contributes to the uniqueness of each individual.

7. Which two main stages of growth and development are most associated with rapid and diverse changes?

8. Which growth and development theorist focuses on how we think and solve problems?

9. Which growth and development theorist focuses on why/how we make moral choices in our behavior?

10. Differentiate nature and nurture as related to Growth & Development potential.

Name: _____

Review

1. Validating cephalocaudal growth patterns, which of the following would develop last during prenatal development?

    a. Legs
    b. Hands
    c. Head
    d. Toes

2. Which of the following is a general principle of human growth and development?

    a. Growth and development proceed from specific to general.
    b. The law of developmental direction proceeds from feet to head.
    c. Development proceeds in a randomized manner.
    d. Development results from the interaction of heredity and environment.

3. Which developmental theorist describes the progression of human cognitive abilities?

    a. Lawrence Kohlberg
    b. Sigmund Freud
    c. Jean Piaget
    d. Erik Eridson

4. The more we interact with our fellow man, the more unique we become.

    a. True
    b. False

Maslow's Hierarchy of Needs

- reaching one's full potential
- pride in accomplishments
- feeling stable and loved
- free from environment risk
- food, water and air.

exposure: either increase or decrease our genetic potential.

Growth
- increase in size and number.

Development
- increase in complexity or Maturation.

Denver II Development Screening Test

Crises - Erikson's psychosocial theory.

Piaget's Theory - cognitive development.

◎ Schema - unit of knowledge.

4 processess
- assimilation
- accommadation
- equilibrium
- disequilibrium

Spiritual Development
James Fowler
Stage 0: Undiffed
Stage 1: Intuitive
Stage 2:

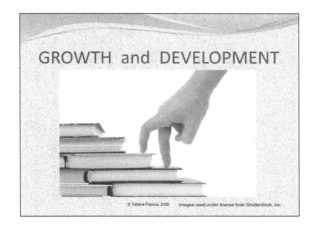

GROWTH and DEVELOPMENT

- OVERVIEW
  - Growth and Development Theory is essential to optimal Nursing care
    - Understanding human response commonalities
    - Individualizing care

- HUMAN RESPONSE COMMONALITIES
  - NEEDS (MASLOW)
    SURVIVAL (food, water, air), SAFETY (free from environmental risks), SECURITY (feeling stable and loved), SELF-ESTEEM (pride in accomplishments), SELF-ACTUALIZATION (reaching one's full potential)
  - BEHAVIOR: PROGRESSIVE DIFFERENTIATION
    The more we interact with others and understand them as well as ourselves, the more UNIQUE we become
  - GROWTH & DEVELOPMENT
    - DIRECTION
    - PROGRESSION
    - PREDICTABILITY

GROWTH and DEVELOPMENT

GROWTH & DEVELOPMENT
- Direction
- Progression
- Predictability

NATURE VS. NURTURE
- Susceptibility (Genetics)
- Exposure (Upbringing)

GROWTH and DEVELOPMENT

- NATURE vs. NURTURE
    Susceptibility vs. Exposure

    - GENETIC INFLUENCES -- DNA (nature)
    -     bone structure, eye color,
            facial features, height

© Alhovik, 2009

ENVIRONMENTAL INFLUENCES (nurture)
    value systems, behavioral patterns

© Liv friis-larsen, 2009

Images used under license from Shutterstock, Inc.

GROWTH and DEVELOPMENT

Physical   Emotional

Nature

Nurture

Cognitive   Socio-Cultural

Courtesy of Patricia Fowler

GROWTH and DEVELOPMENT

GROWTH:
Increase in SIZE or NUMBER
    Characteristics of Human Growth
        Cephalacaudal
        Proximodistal
        Symmetrical
        Sequential but asynchronous

© Sebastian Kaulitzki, 2009

Images used under license from Shutterstock, Inc.

GROWTH and DEVELOPMENT

- DEVELOPMENT
    - GENERAL to SPECIFIC
        - Gross Motor before
        - Fine Motor
        - Both hands catching
            - before one handed
            - catch
    - SIMPLE to COMPLEX
        - Crawling, then Standing, then Walking
        - One word, then phrases, then sentences, then
        - paragraphs

© Jelica Grkic, 2009

Images used under license from Shutterstock, Inc.

GROWTH and DEVELOPMENT

- THEORISTS
    - ERIKSON – PSYCHOSOCIAL

    - PIAGET – COGNITIVE

    - KOHLBERG -- MORAL

GROWTH and DEVELOPMENT

- ERIKSON'S PSYCHOSOCIAL THEORY
    - MAJOR TASKS ASSOCIATED WITH EACH AGE
        - POSITIVE OUTCOME VS. NEGATIVE OUTCOME
            - Trust vs. Mistrust – INFANT
            - Autonomy vs. Shame & Doubt -- TODDLER
            - Initiative vs. Guilt – PRESCHOOL
            - Industry vs. Inferiority – SCHOOL AGE
            - Identity vs. Role confusion – ADOLESCENT
            - Intimacy vs. Isolation – YOUNG ADULT
            - Generativity vs. Stagnation – MIDDLE AGE ADULT
            - Integrity vs. Depression / Despair – ELDER ADULT

GROWTH and DEVELOPMENT
- ERIKSON'S PSYCHOSOCIAL THEORY
  based on
  SIGMUND FREUD'S
  PSYCHOSEXUAL THEORY
  (ID / EGO / SUPEREGO)

© Piko72, 2009

Images used under license from Shutterstock, Inc.

_____
_____
_____
_____
_____
_____
_____
_____

GROWTH and DEVELOPMENT
- JEAN PIAGET'S THEORY ON COGNITION

- CONTINGENT UPON BRAIN
  and NEURAL DEVELOPMENT

  STRONGLY LINKED WITH
  PSYCHOSOCIAL
  DEVELOPMENT

© argus, 2000

Images used under license from Shutterstock, Inc.

_____
_____
_____
_____
_____
_____
_____

GROWTH and DEVELOPMENT
- PIAGET'S THEORY ON COGNITION
  - **REFLEXIVE** (birth to 1 month)

  - **SENSORIMOTOR** (1 month to 2 years)
    - PRIMARY CIRCULAR REACTION, SECONDARY CIRCULAR REACTION, COORDINATION OF SECONDARY SCHEMATA (OBJECT PERMANENCE – 9 -14 months), TERTIARY CIRCULAR REACTION, TRIAL & ERROR, SOLUTION VIA MENTAL COMBINATION

  - **PRE-OPERATIONAL** (2-4 years)
    - PRE-CONCEPTUAL REPRESENTATIONAL THOUGHT (LANGUAGE EXPLOSION)
    - INTUITIVE THOUGHT PROCESSES but with limitation re
      - CAUSE and EFFECT
      - DE-CENTERING

_____
_____
_____
_____
_____
_____
_____

GROWTH and DEVELOPMENT

- PIAGET'S THEORY ON COGNITION
  - **CONCRETE OPERATIONS** (5-12 years)
    - HANDS ON
    - CLASSIFYING, SORTING, RANKING, TIME, CONSERVATION OF MATTER, MEMORY

  - **FORMAL OPERATIONS** (13 ~ ---)
    - ABSTRACT THINKING WITH ABILITY TO HYPOTHESIZE FUTURISTIC AND ALTERNATIVE POSSIBILITIES
      - LIMITATION THROUGHOUT ADOLESCENCE and YOUNG ADULTHOOD related to Inexperience
      - Increases with FLUID INTELLIGENCE that peaks during MIDDLE AGE
      - Enhance by WISDOM that frequently accompanies ELDER YEARS

GROWTH and DEVELOPMENT

- KOHLBERG'S THEORY ON MORALITY

© Liudmila P. Sundikova, 2009

- BASED on research involving males only
  but very similar to Gilligan's research involving females
  (with exception of empathetic caring)

- Very definitely linked with Piaget's theory on Cognition
  Moral choices dependent on ability to process thoughts
  especially related to cause and effect and/or consequences

  Images used under license from Shutterstock, Inc.

GROWTH and DEVELOPMENT

Kohlberg's Theory of Morality

- Addresses individual perspective and potential ability to assume responsibility for actions

- Does not address influences on this perspective:
  - Societal Norms
  - Family and Child rearing values
  - Religious upbringing

GROWTH and DEVELOPMENT

- KOHLBERG'S THEORY OF MORALITY
  - AMORAL (INFANCY)
  - PRE-CONVENTIONAL
    - PUNISHMENT VS. OBEDIENCE
    - INSTRUMENTAL PURPOSE AND EXCHANGE
  - CONVENTIONAL
    - CONFORMITY
    - SOCIAL SYSTEM and DEVELOPMENT of CONSCIENCE
  - POST-CONVENTIONAL
    - SOCIAL CONTRACT and UTILITY
    - UNIVERSAL ETHICAL PRINCIPLES

Pregnancy and First Year of Life

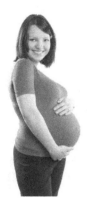

© Lana K, 2009. Used under license from Shutterstock, Inc.

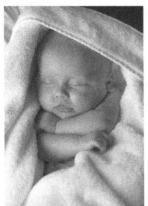

© Wolfgang Amri, 2009. Used under license from Shutterstock, Inc.

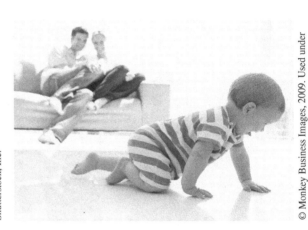

© Monkey Business Images, 2009. Used under license from Shutterstock, Inc.

Objectives

Upon completion of this chapter, the reader should be able to:

1. Relate the impact of parental lifestyles and environmental exposures during pregnancy to the need for planning parenthood in terms of preparing for a healthy baby.
2. Specify the areas evaluated by the Apgar assessment and relate the scores to the overall health of a newborn.
3. Relate the high nutritional and sleep requirement needs of the infant to the rapid rates of growth and development that occur in the first year of life.
4. Describe the developmental status of the sensory and metabolic systems of the infant.
5. Define *anticipatory guidance* and explain how it contributes to growth and development.
6. Describe how infants achieve the psychosocial task of trust and how parents can and should facilitate this process.
7. Relate the role of exposure, experience, and stimulation to the cognitive development of an infant.
8. Describe morality from an infant's perspective.

Key Terms

Anticipatory guidance: health promotion strategies that inform parents and caregivers about expected normals for growth and developmental milestones

Apgar: a health rating system that evaluates the health status of newborns at one minute and five minutes of life

Bonding: an infant's obvious demonstration of comfort and relaxation upon hearing the mother's or father's voice or feeling his/her touch

Developmental milestones: specific behavioral achievements that indicate progression of abilities, for example, rolling over, sitting up, crawling, standing, walking

Object permanence: cognitive ability to know that objects exist even though they may or may not be visibly apparent

Stimulation: exposure to sensory and environmental factors that facilitates cognitive processing

Swaddling: snugly wrapping of infants in a blanket

Weaning: gradual withdrawal from usual practice; during infancy this is the term used for helping infants to withdraw from the breast or bottle and to learn to receive hydration from a cup

Pre-natal Considerations

Growth and development begins *before* conception. Potential parents should be at their healthiest state before considering passing these traits on to their progeny because the health of the parents definitely contributes to the health of the fetus. This means that optimal nutrition and avoidance of drugs (prescription, over the counter [OTC], and/or recreational), avoidance of tobacco products, and moderation of alcohol should be implemented before pregnancy, not after the fact.

In fact, it is in the very early stages of pregnancy in which cell division and so many critical growth and developmental processes occur (in the first trimester). Most often this is happening before parents are even aware that they have conceived.

Some of the more common contributors to problems occurring during pregnancy are blunt force trauma; chemical exposure to radiation and pesticides (DDT); medications and/or recreational drugs; alcohol; vaccine-preventable communicable diseases like rubella and varicella; sexually transmitted disease such as gonorrhea, syphilis, and chlamydia; serious infections like toxoplasmosis (from undercooked meat); and chronic disease such as diabetes and heart disease. Most, if not all, of these factors can be minimized through healthy lifestyle choices of the parents. Blood type incompatibility (Rh factor) is another factor that may impact negatively on the health of the fetus but this can readily be identified and treated if and when the pregnant female receives early prenatal care.

Another factor definitely contributing to the health of the fetus is how well the pregnancy was planned. Unplanned or unanticipated pregnancies very often result in unwanted pregnancies. These unanticipated pregnancies, as a result of careless, indiscriminate sexual encounters, rape, and/or miscalculated protective, preventive or barrier methodology, can impact dramatically on the health of the fetus and can also impact very negatively on infants and young children. This unfortunately results too often in failure to thrive and also in the increased risk of physical and emotional abuse.

Teenage pregnancies are particularly vulnerable to problems. Not only are most of these pregnancies unplanned, but the situation exists when children are bearing and rearing children. The teenage body, though mature enough to conceive and sustain a pregnancy, is usually NOT in the best of health. Adolescents, generally speaking, do not have optimal nutrition and/or adequate sleep patterns. Adding the potential for tobacco, alcohol, and/or drug experimentation and sexually transmitted disease only further complicates the issue. Then when one considers the instability of financial wherewithal, and age-related absence of maturity and accountability, it becomes evident that adolescent pregnancies are most often determined to be high-risk pregnancies.

Infancy: Birth to One Year of Age

Assessments

Despite potentially adverse conditions, somehow most babies are born relatively healthy. Immediately upon their arrival into this earthly existence, health care providers evaluate the health status of infants by using an assessment tool known as the **Apgar.** The Apgar assessment is a quick and easy rating of color

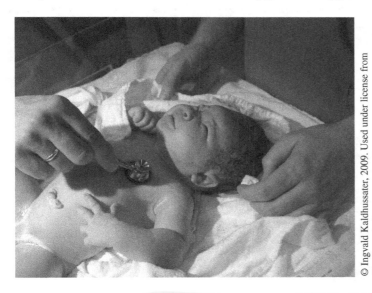

© Ingvald Kaldhussater, 2009. Used under license from Shutterstock, Inc.

(the pinker the better), heart rate (fast and regular is good), reflex irritability (the quickness of response to tactile stimuli), muscle tone (how tightly and/or forcefully they move muscles as opposed to having flaccid or limp movements), and how well their lungs take in air. This evaluation assessment of a 0, 1, or 2 in these five categories is summed up for a rating at one minute after birth and again at at five minutes after birth. Obviously the closer to 10 the Apgar rating is, the healthier the baby.

Infants are also assessed for the ability to hear because hearing is fully

developed at birth and is essential to bonding and learning to interact with the world. The infant's eyes are checked for infection but not for vision since vision is not fully developed until around six years of age.

Infants are also assessed for their ability to suck. Sucking is obviously necessary for infants to intake the nutrients that their bodies need. When the sucking reflex is weak, infants may need special nipples and/or IV fluids to sustain their nutritional needs. Sucking is also a comfort need. This is an argument FOR pacifiers.

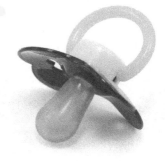

© Adrov Andriy, 2009. Used under license from Shutterstock, Inc.

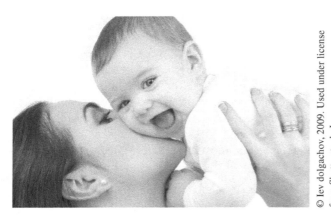

© Iev dolgachov, 2009. Used under license from Shutterstock, Inc.

Infants are also assessed for **bonding**. Bonding is a term that describes a natural connectedness that exists between a newborn and his/her mother or father or primary caregiver. This is evaluated by the spontaneity of comfort exhibited by the infant when hearing the mother's or father's voice or feeling their touch. This is also assessed by the natural molding of the infant's body to the mother's or father's shape so that they just seem to fit. Absence of bonding has been associated with failure to thrive.

Newborn infants are also weighed and measured and evaluated against gestational age standards. Most newborns weigh 7 to 9 pounds and are 18 to 22 inches in length but there is a wide range of normal depending on the parent's genetic potential. Infants weighing less than 5 pounds are assessed as low birth weight and often considered to be at higher risk.

Growth is rapid during the first year of life. Even though it is common for newborns to lose up to 10% of their birth weight in the first few days of life (related to the stress of coming into this world), they usually rapidly gain this weight back and will continue to gain 5 to 7 ounces per week for the first 6 weeks. Generally speaking, most infants will double their birth weight by 6 months of age and triple their birth weight by one year. Similarly infants will increase their birth length in the first year of life by 1½ times, that is, an infant measuring 20 inches at birth will likely be 30 inches long at one year.

Growth Requirements

To meet the body requirements to sustain the rapid growth rate of infants, lots of calories (110–120 calories/kg or 200 ml/kg) are required. And because of the limited capacity of the digestive system, this means that most infants require feeding 3 to 4 ounces of liquid every 3 to 4 hours. Breast feeding, because of the rich nutrients and maternal antibodies, is usually recommended but, when this cannot be offered, infant formulas fortified with iron are quite adequate.

Infants are usually weaned from the breast or bottle before their first birthday. *Weaning* is a term referring to helping the infant to withdraw from the breast or bottle. In so doing, the infant learns a new way of receiving hydration. Most infants are weaned to a small cup with a lip. The lip on the cup helps to prevent spills but also allows infants to close their mouth down over it to be more akin to clamping down on a nipple. Infants then progress from a cup with a lip to a cup without a lip and use of a straw.

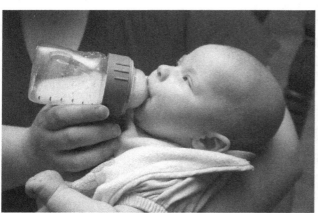

© Johanna Goodyear, 2009. Used under license from Shutterstock, Inc.

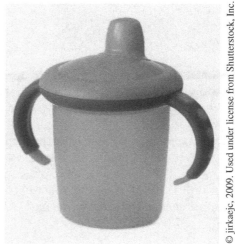

© jirkaejc, 2009. Used under license from Shutterstock, Inc.

The digestive system of an infant is too immature to process solid food (even soft or pureed food) until about 6 months of age. When solid (pureed) foods are first given, they should be introduced one at a time to evaluate digestive tolerance as well as the infant's absence of allergic response. Based on the ease of digestive processes, the following sequence is usually recommended. Cereals should be started first, then vegetables, then fruits. Meats should not be introduced until around 9 months of age. If digestively tolerated, soft and/or pureed table foods can also be introduced between 9 and 12 months of age.

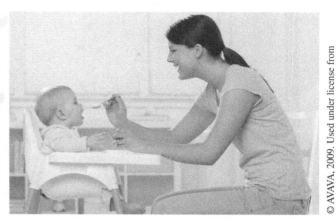

© AVAVA, 2009. Used under license from Shutterstock, Inc.

Because they are growing so rapidly, infants require a tremendous amount of sleep. Most newborns sleep 18–22 hours per day, waking only to be fed and/or changed. Common household noises generally do not disturb the sleep of infants so there is no need to create a noise free environment. By 4 months of age, infants have a greater stomach capacity and can therefore sleep in longer intervals but they still sleep approximately 16 hours/day. By their first birthday, most infants require 12 hours of sleep/day and this includes 1–2 nap times of 1–2 hours.

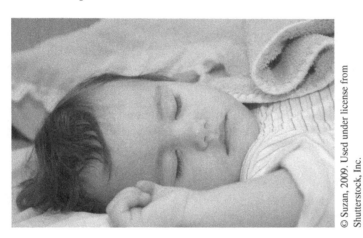

© Suzan, 2009. Used under license from Shutterstock, Inc.

What do you think?

Has the risk for sudden infant death syndrome (SIDS) been minimized by the practice of placing infants on their backs for sleep? What researched evidence exists about this practice?

During infancy there is a danger of Sudden Infant Death Syndrome (SIDS). This is a term applied to crib deaths from "unknown causes." Research indicates that the small nasal passage plus the inability of the infant to turn their head from side to side may contribute to accidental suffocation when babies are in a prone position. For this reason, it is recommended that infants always be placed on their backs or sides for sleep.

Appearance

Newborns, though often described as adorable and beautiful, generally have characteristics that defy these descriptions. For the most part, babies have extremely large heads that may be conical in shape from passage through the birth canal. In addition, their chest circumference is as large as their head circumference and their arms and legs are extremely short. This disproportionate being, in reality, could only be beautiful to the eyes of the beholders (their loving parents and relatives). But as stated in the growth and development overview, we know that, in time, the infant's body will grow and develop to become more proportionate.

Actions

Newborns are born with certain spontaneous, reflexive behaviors that include rooting, sucking, and grasping. A gentle wisp of a touch on the cheek will cause them to turn their head to the direction of the touch—this is the rooting reflex and is particularly useful to the infant to help them find the mother's breast or the nipple on the bottle of formula. Newborns are also born with a built-in need and ability to suck. This allows them to immediately obtain nutrients and begin their growth processes. Holding a finger at the base of the palm of their hands will result in their opening of the fingers and grasping onto your finger. This, too, is reflexive behavior and does not mean that they are purposely holding on to your finger. The moro reflex is apparent when both arms and legs respond with a forward jerk when there is a loud noise.

Did you know?

Did you know that without hearing infants will not learn to talk? They must first hear the sounds before they begin to imitate them.

Did you know that most babies learn to say "DaDa" before they say "MaMa"? This is because the d's are much easier to articulate than the m's—and it has nothing to do with favoritism.

The sensory system in newborns has varied levels of maturation. The ability to feel, hear, taste, and smell is completely developed and functional at full capacity at birth. The ability to taste is evident in the infant's eager intake of breast milk or formula milk. The feeling of touch is evident in the rooting reflex described above and in the infant's ability to respond to stimuli (both painful and pleasurable) as evaluated with the Apgar ratings. The sense of hearing is evident in the response to loud noise (jerking reaction) or a calming expression with soft, gentle sounds. Because hearing is so essential to communication and to the intake of stimuli, hearing tests are now performed on every newborn so that any deficit can be carefully remedied as early as possible. Smell is completely developed in the newborn as well and is the mechanism by which most infants recognize their mothers, fathers, and caregivers.

Vision is the one sense that is not developed well at birth. Vision, at birth, is extremely nearsighted and very nondiscriminatory because it is for the most part non-focused. Vision actually does not become binocular and selective until around 6 months of age. Until then, most visual images are blurs at best. And vision is not fully developed until around age 6.

In terms of body systems management, these too are varied. Temperature regulation is not well developed. Infants do not have the ability to sweat or to shiver in response to temperature extremes, so caregivers must maintain environmental temperature and clothing adjustments for them. This does not mean that infants need to be 10 degrees warmer than anyone else in the room.

Swaddling is a common practice in the care of the newborn. Swaddling simply means that the infant is enclosed in a snug wrapping. This does not allow for air drafts on any part of the body and is supposedly also akin to the feeling of being snugly enclosed that was experienced in utero. Therefore, it is assumed that this is a comforting feeling for the newborn. Evidence that this is so is recognizing that most infants do in fact, eat, sleep, and appear more relaxed when they have been swaddled. But since infants need to have the freedom to move arms and legs freely, swaddling should not be extended beyond the first few weeks of life.

Body System Development

Most body systems are not fully developed at birth. For example, the kidneys are not yet developed sufficiently to concentrate urine resulting in the need for frequent diaper changes. The digestive processes are also immature so that the dietary intake must be limited to liquids (preferably breast milk or formula and water only). The intestinal tract does not yet have the ability to reabsorb water, so the result is loose stools. The lungs are very small and inefficient so the respiratory rate is fast and the depth of the respirations is shallow. Similarly, the heart is small, causing the heart rate to be rapid.

There is tremendous growth and maturation of the brain not only during infancy, but during the first 12 years of life. Even though the infant's head

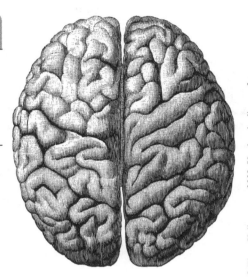

© Elena Kalistratova, 2009. Used under license from Shutterstock, Inc.

appears extremely large, it must be noted that there are gaps in the skull. These are known as fontanels: a quadrilateral "soft spot" toward the front of the skull and a triangular "soft spot" in the posterior section of the skull. The posterior fontanel usually closes between the ages of 2 and 4 months but the anterior fontanel may remain at least partially open up until 18 months of age. These fontanels allow room for the brain to grow and become larger. Not only does the brain become larger, but it also becomes far more developed. At birth, the axons and dendrites of the complex neural system are few and far between and there is essentially no myelin on the neural pathways. Between birth and 6 years of age, this becomes a myriad of neural plexus systems.

Need for Stimulation

Just as the infant body requires food and hydration and sleep to grow, the infant's body and brain also requires stimulation. Infants need to have freedom of movement, exposure to bright and differentiating colors, exposure to variations in sound (both in pitch and volume and tempo), and the ability to experience the different tastes and feel of textures. Above all, infants need to have the opportunity not only to be exposed to these things but the opportunity to explore these things in a safe environment.

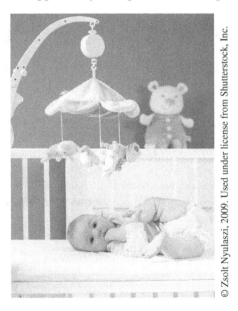

© Zsolt Nyulaszi, 2009. Used under license from Shutterstock, Inc.

Exposure and experience equals **stimulation**. Stimulation is necessary to encourage the brain to make progressive complex arborizations of the dendrites, to increase the vascularization of certain anatomical structures of the brain (e.g., images associated with vision), and to increase the process of myelinization.

Providing stimulation to infants is not as simple as it seems. It is one thing to allow and encourage infants to experience the world; it is another whole realm that also requires parents to be forever vigilant, that is, available and accessible for constant supervision. Safety is critical during infancy because infants not only do not have bodily control of movement, but they obviously do not have cognitive discernment of factors that may harm them. Infant deaths are all too often associated with suffocation, aspiration, falls, drowning, poisoning, and burns. The number one cause of accidental death during infancy is motor vehicle accident. This, by the way, is the number one cause of accidental death for individuals of all ages.

Anticipatory Guidance

Experts in the field have determined that there are pertinent holistic health strategies that can and should be strongly promoted to maximize potentials and to minimize risks during certain stages of Growth and Development. These strategies, when provided to parents and to caregivers are commonly known as **anticipatory guidance**. Anticipatory guidance just simply means that when the potentials as well as the risks associated with normal **developmental milestones** in growth and development stages are known and anticipated, then there is a much better chance that these potentials and risks can be maximized or minimized as indicated.

Examples of infant developmental milestones for anticipatory guidance:

Age	Gross Motor Milestone Expectations	Fine Motor Milestone Expectations
2 months	Lifts head when prone	Fading grasp reflex
3–4 months	Turns from side to side	Holds rattle placed in hand
4–6 months	Rolls from back to front; front to back	Plays with feet; holds bottle
7–8 months	Sits; crawls	Transfers objects from one hand to other
9–10 months	Pulls self to standing	Shows hand preference
11–12 months	Walks; can sit from standing position	Feeds self well with fingers; beginning to use large utensils

Remember this.

When infants fail to achieve anticipated developmental milestones, there is need for thorough evaluation and referral. The **Denver II** is a simple to administer assessment tool to identify developmental delays and should be used at every Well Baby Check-up. This Assessment is mandatory under the Texas Steps Medicaid requirement and assesses progress in the following areas:

- *Self-help skills* like dressing and eating + Psychosocial skills like sharing
- *Sensory abilities* (this includes hearing, vision and language)
- *Fine Motor skills* like using thumb finger grasp
- *Gross Motor skills* like sitting, crawling, standing, walking

The Denver II is frequently administered at the same time as the Well Baby Check-up with the pediatrician at 2, 4, 6 and 12 months. These are important check-ups to make sure that the infants are progressing physiologically as well as developmentally. This also makes a great opportunity to keep the infants on the recommended vaccine schedule.

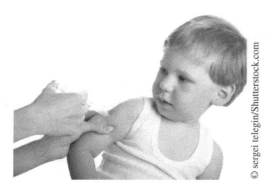

© sergei telegin/Shutterstock.com

At birth and for the next 2–3 months, infants are protected from many infectious diseases because they have the bonus of maternal antibodies that have been transferred to them in utero. But this passive immunity does not persist. So infants need to receive vaccines to build their own antibody resistance. Vaccines required for infants include hepatitis A, hepatitis B, measles, mumps, rubella, varicella, polio, pertussis, diphtheria, tetanus, hemophilus influenza type B, pneumonia, rotovirus, and flu.

Even though repeatedly proven to be false, there have been some reports that supposedly linked vaccines with autism. This caused many parents to refuse to have their infants vaccinated.

This is potentially very dangerous for these children since they have no immunity and it is also extremely bad for the whole country because diseases that have been essentially eradicated are re-surfacing. Parents need to have their children vaccinated.

Other areas of anticipatory guidance include information relating to psychosocial, cognitive, and language skills; the need for scheduled immunizations; and the need to take special precautions relating to car seat safety, sleeping positioning, household protective measures relating to poisons and toxic agents, and risks relating to choking on small objects.

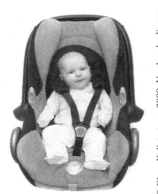

© Elena Kalistratova, 2009. Used under license from Shutterstock, Inc.

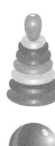

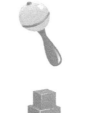

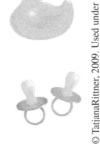

© TatjanaRittner, 2009. Used under license from Shutterstock, Inc.

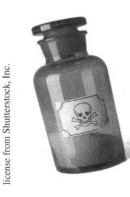

© jirkaejc, 2009. Used under license from Shutterstock, Inc.

Developmental Theories

Erik Erikson's Psychosocial Theory, Piaget's Cognitive Theory, and Kohlberg's Theory of Morality will be used as the bases for learning more about these anticipated needs. Please remember that infants are totally dependent upon their caregivers for food, diapering, sleep, and comfort. Since infants do not have the ability to obtain these things for themselves, they totally rely on their caregivers to take care of them. So, when caregivers respond to needs in a prompt and consistent manner, infants learn to trust that their needs will be satisfied and that they are in safe hands. When they are left hungry, wet, and in a stage of discomfort repeatedly, they learn NOT to trust others.

In accordance with Erikson's theory, all individuals need to achieve and sustain self-esteem. This is accomplished when they resolve the "crisis" associated with their stage of development. And according to Erikson, accomplishment of tasks at subsequent stages can only be achieved when the crisis task is achieved in the current stage. This means that infants who do not learn to trust during infancy will have great difficulty achieving the tasks of autonomy, initiative, industry, identity, intimacy, generativity, or integrity.

Infants learn who they are from the reaction of others to them. They recognize that, even though they are totally dependent upon others, they are also uniquely separate from others. They learn to desire affection but also how to adjust to expectations. So, can infants become spoiled? Of course, but they can also learn some degree of restraint and limitation if caregivers respond to them consistently. For example, just because an infant is crying does not mean that they need to be picked up and held. Do infants like to be held? Of course, but they should not be held all the time. Often babies cry just because they feel insecure. This does not necessarily mean that they need to be held. So parents can talk or sing to them or just pat them on the back to let them know that they are nearby without necessarily always picking infants up. This helps infants to learn trust and separateness and minimizes the risk for them to become spoiled.

Infants also learn to differentiate live versus inanimate objects. They know that movement and sound from mobiles are very different from the touch and voice of their mother or the nuzzling and barking of the family dog. Infants are also learning about equilibrium in the beginning stages of bodily control (balancing arms and legs to change positions) and balancing their needs versus their wants.

So what are infants thinking about? Or more importantly, HOW are they thinking about it? That is, how are they processing information and what are they doing with it? Thinking, or cognition, according to Jean Piaget (1950), is a process involving exposure to new experiences or information that causes us to rethink. Re-thinking involves a complex adaptation through assimilation and accommodation so that the new experience and/or exposure "fits."

For the first 2 to 4 months of life, infants are in a "reflexive" stage. During this stage movements are neuromuscularly controlled rather than purposefully controlled. Sucking is probably the most prominent reflexive action of an infant. No one has taught them or shown them how to suck but they do this spontaneously. Another reflexive activity is grasping. Infants will close their fingers around yours if you lightly move your finger from the base of the palm of the infant to the bottom of their fingers. The rooting reflex is demonstrated by seeing that the infant spontaneously turns to the direction of stroking on their cheek. This is apparent when trying to get the infant to nurse. When infants are held upright and facing away from the holder, they will lift and move their feet in a climbing or dancing fashion. This is known as the dancing reflex. This rooting, sucking, grasping and dancing reflex, as described above, are typical of this reflexive stage.

Piaget labels the next stage as "sensorimotor." During this stage, infants actually begin to process information purposefully but it begins with use of their senses (what they see, hear, taste, smell, and feel). According to Piaget's Sensorimotor Stage, there are five stages: primary circular reaction, secondary circular reaction, coordination of secondary schemata, tertiary circular reaction and solutions by mental combinations. In the primary circular reaction stage, infants merely react to something in their environment. For example, they may see a spinning motion when they accidentally touched a part of the mobile that was over the crib. So they think, "Hey, that's pretty neat." If and when this occurs again, they start paying attention to how and when this occurred. When this happens, they think, "I want to make that happen again" and they try to re-create the action. This is "secondary circular reaction." After repeated efforts, memory serves them well and they remember how this occurs. This now becomes the stage of "coordination of secondary schemata" and progresses to tertiary circular reaction and solutions by mental combinations. (Review these stages in the G & D Overview chapter.)

Object permanence is a major factor during the coordination of secondary schemata stage. This concept describes the ability to remember that an object or person exists even though it may or may not be immediately visible. This is when infants know that what is out of sight is NOT necessarily out of mind. Parents can no longer hide something behind their back and think that the infant will lose interest. Nor will they accept readily the distraction of a babysitter. They now know that Mom and Dad are truly not at home. This phenomenon usually occurs between 9 and 14 months of age and is generally speaking a very traumatic stage for most young parents. When it is apparent that infants are in this stage, parents are encouraged to initially take short trips away from the house and always with a quick return. This helps reassure the infant that the parent is still present even if not seen and it helps them to better trust that the parent will return.

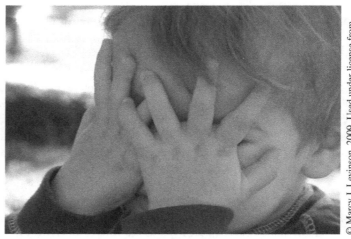

Learning language is also a key component of cognition. Connecting the recognition of a familiar term with the use of certain objects helps the infants to learn and imitate words. Calling objects by their correct name is strongly encouraged to help infants to learn it right the first time rather than having to unlearn and relearn later.

According to Lawrence Kohlberg (1969), morality is really a non-issue during the infancy stage. Morality, as described by Kohlberg, is classified by the degree or extent to which a person's cognitive ability allows them to perceive an action. Therefore, since an infant has not had the opportunity to process an extensive amount of information to determine if it is good or bad, they really cannot be assessed as moral or not moral. Kohlberg's Amoral Stage, therefore, does not mean that infants choose to act without morals; it simply means that they have not yet experienced life enough to even have morals. For most infants, "if it feels good, do it" is the only morality that exists.

Summary

While infancy can and should be an absolutely fascinating experience, this is unfortunately not always the case. Just because individuals are capable of reproducing does not make them good parents and it is a sad fact that not all parents have good parenting skills. When there is an absence of bonding between mother/father and infant, many infants fail to thrive, that is, they do not grow and/or develop as they should. This also occurs when infants are abused (physically or mentally) or neglected. Parents need to have appropriate expectations of their infant, competence and confidence in parenting skills, and a strong sense of their own self-esteem. This means that parents must balance their own personal needs and wants with the stress and responsibility of being a caregiver.

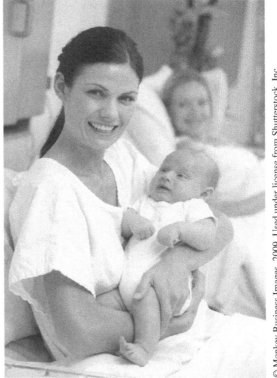

© Monkey Business Images, 2009. Used under license from Shutterstock, Inc.

Infants, by nature of their immature bodies and brains and immune systems, are extremely vulnerable to injury, illness, and/or disease. This is why parents and caregivers at all times need to be providers and protectors. But, even when parenting skills are optimal, illnesses occur. The most common health problems associated with infancy are in the respiratory, gastrointestinal, and dermatological systems. These conditions, though not addressed in this text, will be discussed in great detail later in the nursing curriculum.

References

Erikson, E. H. (1968) *Childhood and society* (35th anniversary ed.). New York: Norton.

Kohlberg, L. (1969). *The philosophy of moral development: Vol. 1.* San Francisco: Harper & Row.

Piaget, J. (1950). *The psychology of intelligence.* London: Routledge and Kegan Paul.

Reflection

In the space below, reflect on your personal experience with an infant and share how this experience either supports the theory about this stage of development or contradicts it.

Assignment

The form below is an example of how to create a future study sheet. Please feel free to add additional information and know that you will be expected to complete a form like this for each of the ages discussed in the next chapters.

Growth and Development Guide

	Physical Traits	Physical Abilities	Psychosocial Task (Erikson)	Evidence of How Achieved	Evidence of Non-Achievement	Cognitive Ability (Piaget)	Evidence of Achievement	Moral Capability (Kohlberg)	Evidence of Achievement
Infant (Birth—15 months)	Short arms and legs; Flat nose; Teeth eruption: bottom 2 first @ 4–6 mos. Limited vision but full sense of hearing and smell	Roll over by 4 mos.; Sit by 5 mos.; Crawl by 7 mos.; Stand by 9 mos.; Walk by 12 mos. Babbling and beginning speech sounds: DaDa & MaMa	Trust vs. Mistrust	Bonding & showing comfort when held; Responding to parent voice	Frequent cry Non-responsive to parent voice Awkward positioning when held	Reflexive Sensorimotor Primary, Secondary & Coordination of secondary schemata Tertiary Reaction Solution via mental combinations	See, Feel, Touch, Taste, Smell Everything Explore use of toys	Amoral	"If it feels good, do it"

Name: _____

Study Guide for
Pregnancy and First Year of Life

1. Describe the physical/physiological characteristics of infants in terms of heart rate, respirations, temperature regulation, nutrition and sleep requirements and growth parameters.

2. Describe the sensory (5 senses) capabilities of the infant.

3. Explain how these senses are used to master Piaget's first stage of cognitive development.

4. Describe what fontanels are, where they are located, what purpose they serve and how long they persist.

5. Define bonding, give at least one example of how it would be evident and explain how this relates to infant survival.

6. Describe the time frame and sequence for introducing solid (pureed) food to infants and explain why this sequence is recommended.

7. Explain why a pacifier is a good thing for infants

8. Define weaning and explain how and when an infant should be weaned from the bottle.

9. Explain how an infant develops trust in his/her caregiver and differentiate this from "spoiling" the infant.

10. Explain why infants are designated as "amoral" and explain exactly what this means.

Name: _____

Review

1. By age 1, a baby who weighed 7 pounds at birth and was 20 inches long will now weigh approximately _____ pounds and be about _____ inches in length.
   a. 14...40
   b. 12...30
   c. 21...30
   d. 30...30

2. In order for an infant to develop the psychosocial task of TRUST, there must be
   a. enforcement of limit setting as early as 4 months of age to prepare for the real world.
   b. consistent and prompt response to their needs by parents and caregivers.
   c. reciprocal trust exhibited by parents and caregivers.
   d. constant attention and cuddling.

3. Which of the following is indicative of ineffective bonding between mother and baby?
   a. sustained eye contact between mother and baby
   b. mother calling the baby by name
   c. molding of baby's body to mother's when being held
   d. infant irritability even when being picked up

4. Babies should be weaned from the bottle or breast by 6 months of age.
   a. True
   b. False

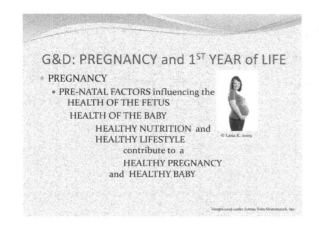

G&D: PREGNANCY and 1ST YEAR of LIFE

- PREGNANCY
  - PRE-NATAL FACTORS influencing the
    HEALTH OF THE FETUS
    HEALTH OF THE BABY
    HEALTHY NUTRITION and
    HEALTHY LIFESTYLE
      contribute to a
        HEALTHY PREGNANCY
        and HEALTHY BABY

© Lana K. 2009

Images used under license from Shutterstock, Inc.

G&D: PREGNANCY and 1ST YEAR of LIFE

HEALTHY PREGNANCY
   Need to avoid alcohol, tobacco, chemical
exposure, (X-ray) medications including over-the-counter
and illegal substances and the potential for acquiring
communicable and/or sexually transmitted disease

PLANNED PREGNANCY = WANTED PREGNANCY
   with COMMITMENT

   MAJOR CONCERNS with TEEN PREGNANCIES

PRE-NATAL CARE ESSENTIAL

EVALUATION for Rh factor / risks

G&D: PREGNANCY and 1ST YEAR of LIFE

First moments of life evaluated by **APGAR**
      1 minute and 5 minute evaluations:
   Assessment of
      heart rate,
      respiratory rate,
      color,
      reflex response to stimuli and
      muscle tone
      ** Closer to 10 the better**

   Assessment for Hearing
   Assessment for PKU *

   Infants are also assessed for their
   ability to suck (essential for nutrient
   intake)and for the mother-baby
   favorable interaction known as
   BONDING

© Monkey Business Images, 2009

© Adrov Andriy, 2009

© lev dolgachov, 2009

Images used under license from Shutterstock, Inc.

G&D: PREGNANCY and 1ST YEAR of LIFE

ASSESSMENT OF HEIGHT AND WEIGHT
  WEIGHT: *Double birth weight by 6 months; Triple by 1 year*

GROWTH REQUIREMENTS
  INFANT NUTRITION
  Frequent feedings due to small gastric system
      BREAST FEEDING IS ALWAYS BEST
          IMMUNE FACTORS (maternal antibodies)
          BONDING
      FORMULA FEEDING
          Good but allergies possible
      SOLID FOODS
      not until 6 months, then
          one at a time for one week
          in following sequence
          Cereals,
          Vegetables,
          Fruit,
          Meat (9-12 months)

© AVAVA, 2009
Images used under license from Shutterstock, Inc.

- decrease risk of obesity
- saving money.
- decrease risk of cancer.

G&D: PREGNANCY and 1ST YEAR of LIFE

- *WEANING*
  - From Bottle to Cup (6 months–1 yr)
    - Important for future dentition
  - SLEEP -- 18-22 hrs. /day initially
      required for GROWTH
      decreases to 12 hrs by 1 year but
      still need afternoon nap
      Infants should be placed on back when
      sleeping to minimize potential for
      •Sudden Infant Death syndrome (SIDS)•

© Johanna Goodyear, 2009
© Jirkaejc, 2009
© Suzan, 2009
Images used under license from Shutterstock, Inc.

triple their size.

NO co-bedding.

G&D: PREGNANCY and 1ST YEAR of LIFE

- Characteristic Appearance of Newborn
  - Large head, short limbs

- *Fontanels* on skull to allow for
    brain growth but also leaves the
    infant vulnerable to brain damage
    when beaten or shaken
      Anterior fontanel open up till 18 months of age
      Posterior fontanel closes between 2-4 months

© Elena Kalistratova, 2009
Images used under license from Shutterstock.

fontanels are a great
assessment.

G&D: PREGNANCY and 1ST YEAR of LIFE

Actions
Reflexes
- Rooting (turning toward cheek stimuli -- seeking source of feeding)
- Moro (startle) – both arms, both legs jerking in response to loud noise
- Grasp reflex – encircling object when palm is stroked upward
- Dance reflex: moving feet in dancing motion

G&D: PREGNANCY and 1ST YEAR of LIFE

- Newborn Senses
  - Hearing, taste, smell and touch senses completely intact
  - (Vision very limited)– progressively improves in distance perception from 6 months of age up until 6 years of age
  - Temperature regulation very poor (no ability to sweat and/shiver.) Swaddling provides warmth and security.

G&D: PREGNANCY and 1ST YEAR of LIFE

Body System Development
Immature lungs, kidneys, digestive tract,

Brain (not fully developed until age 12) – concern regarding shaken baby syndrome

© Elena Kalistratova, 2009

Images used under license from Shutterstock, Inc.

G&D: PREGNANCY and 1ST YEAR of LIFE

- Newborn Needs
  - *Stimulation*
    - Colorful, moving objects
    - Sound: music, talking, objects that make sounds
    - Touch: holding, cuddling = bonding
  - *Non-confining space* in which to move and explore

G&D: PREGNANCY and 1ST YEAR of LIFE

- Newborn Needs
  - **Safety**
    - Car Safety seats
    - No dangling tablecloths and no breakable objects within reach
    - *Anything that can go in an infant's mouth, will –*
      - Nothing potentially poisonous should be accessible
      - No objects with small detachable parts
      - Nothing plastic
    - SUPERVISION at ALL TIMES – don't turn your back!

G&D: PREGNANCY and 1ST YEAR of LIFE

ANTICIPATORY GUIDANCE

Gross Motor Milestone Expectations Sequence
- **Lifts head when prone (tummy)**
- **Turns from side to side**
- **Rolls from back to front; front to back**
- **Sits; crawls**
- **Pulls self to standing**
- **Walks**
- **Can sit from standing position**

G&D: PREGNANCY and 1ST YEAR of LIFE

Fine Motor Milestone Expectations
- Fading grasp reflex
- Holds rattle placed in hand
- Plays with feet
- Holds bottle
- Transfers objects from one hand to the other
- Shows hand preference
- Feeds self well with fingers
- Begins using large utensils

G&D: PREGNANCY and 1ST YEAR of LIFE

• PARENTING SKILLS
ANTICIPATORY GUIDANCE
- awareness of developmental milestones and having realistic expectations
  - Relating to physical and psychomotor abilities
  - Relating to psychosocial interactions
  - Relating to cognitive and language development
  - Relating to behavioral expectations

G&D: PREGNANCY and 1ST YEAR of LIFE

PARENTING SKILLS
Related to UNREALISTIC EXPECTATIONS
- Results in Parental / Infant frustration
- Results in Parental neglect which results in infant injury from normal explorations
- Results in Parental abuse resulting in infant massive injury
  - Shaken baby syndrome / broken bones

G&D: PREGNANCY and 1ST YEAR of LIFE

INFANT DEVELOPMENTAL ASSESSMENT

When infants fail to achieve anticipated developmental milestones, there is a need for thorough evaluation and referral.

G&D: PREGNANCY and 1ST YEAR of LIFE

INFANT ASSESSMENT

The **Denver II** is a simple to administer assessment tool to identify developmental delays and should be used at every Well Baby Check-up. This Assessment is mandatory under the Texas Steps Medicaid requirement and assesses progress in the following areas:

- *Self-help skills* like dressing and eating + Psychosocial skills like sharing
- *Sensory abilities* (this includes hearing, vision and language)
- *Fine Motor skills* like using thumb finger grasp
- *Gross Motor skills* like sitting, crawling, standing, walking

G&D: PREGNANCY and 1ST YEAR of LIFE

INFANT ASSESSMENT

- **Well Baby Check –up** (pediatrician)
  - 2, 4, 6, 12 months
- **Vaccines:**
  hepatitis A, hepatitis B, measles, mumps, rubella, varicella, polio, pertussis, diphtheria, tetanus, hemophilus influenza type B, pneumonia, rotovirus, and flu.

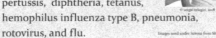

Images used under license from Shutterstock, Inc.

G&D: PREGNANCY and 1ST YEAR of LIFE

- INFANT PSYCHOSOCIAL TASK (ERIKSON)
  - **TRUST**
    - Gained by caregivers responding to basic needs (hunger, diapering, comfort, security, temperature variations, stimulation) in a *caring, consistent manner*
    - Evidenced by following caregivers voice, reaching out eagerly for caregiver, resting comfortably in arms of caregiver, smiling with delight when caregiver approaches
  - MIS-TRUST
    - Gained by inconsistency and/or non-caring attitude
    - Evidenced by indifference to nearness of caregiver and general mal-content

G&D: PREGNANCY and 1ST YEAR of LIFE

- Can Infants be spoiled?
  - Babies cry when they want something. Because they cannot yet speak, this is the only way infants have to communicate. But a few minutes of crying will not cause emotional trauma.
  - Yet if parents hold their infants all the time and never allow them to experience small tastes of delayed gratification, they can become dependent upon that instant gratification and this is a hard habit to break

G&D: PREGNANCY and 1ST YEAR of LIFE

- COGNITION
  - Reflexive stage: 1-4 months
  - Sensorimotor
    - Primary Circular Reaction – recognizing a familiar visual object and/or recognizing a familiar audible sound
    - Secondary Circular Reaction – attempt to create visual object and/or sound (cry for Mom or bottle / bring thumb to mouth to suck

G&D: PREGNANCY and 1ST YEAR of LIFE

- COGNITION (Object Permanence)
  - Coordination of Secondary Schemata
    - recognizing that one action results in a predictable response and remembering it
  - Recognizing that out of sight does not mean "not there"
  - No more hiding objects behind back – they will be found
  - Difficulties with Mom and Dad leaving baby with babysitter – infant knows they are somewhere and are just ignoring them

Images used under license from Shutterstock, Inc.

G&D: PREGNANCY and 1ST YEAR of LIFE

- COGNITION – LANGUAGE
  - Connecting words (sounds) with objects and repeating
  - Important to use correct enunciation
    - Baby talk NOT encouraged

- MORALITY (KOHLBERG)
  - AMORAL – If it feels good, do it!
    - Infants do not have the cognitive ability to discern right from wrong!
    - Infants do have the ability to know what gives them positive responses and what does not.

Toddler (Age 1–3)

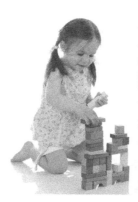

© Dagmara Ponikiewska, 2009. Used under license from Shutterstock, Inc.

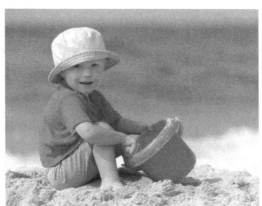

© Trutta, 2009. Used under license from Shutterstock, Inc.

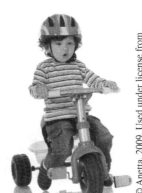

© Anetta, 2009. Used under license from Shutterstock, Inc.

Objectives

Upon completion of this chapter, the reader should be able to:

1. Describe the physical and physiologic characteristics of a toddler.
2. Compare and contrast the growth rate of a toddler to that of an infant and relate to nutritional and sleep requirements.
3. Describe the role of play in helping the toddler to achieve autonomy.
4. Identify the major tasks involved in achieving autonomy.
5. Describe the parental challenges during the toddler age period.

Key Terms

Childproofing: removing objects considered potentially harmful to young children

Finger foods: foods capable of being picked up with hands and eaten without the need for utensils

Food jag: preferring only one type of food repeatedly over a period of time

Parallel play: play environment characterized by several children playing independently in the same location without communication or interaction

Waddle: walking like a duck; moving almost as much from side to side as going forward

Toddler Physical Characteristics

Around the time that an infant reaches one year of age, the body proportions shift. Now the chest is larger than the head, and the limbs (arms and legs) are growing faster than the trunk. Toddlers often seem to **waddle** when they walk because they need to sustain a wide stance to balance their protruding bellies on their relatively short legs. There is a thickening of the skin epithelium which makes them less vulnerable to rashes and surface injuries.

Another physical characteristic of toddlers is that they now have up to 16 teeth. With teeth, toddlers have the capability to chew and to bite and have the increased potential for dental caries. The increased capacity to chew means that toddlers can ingest more complex foods such as apples and ground meat. And because the stomach is larger and the digestive processes are more developed, they tend to eat less frequently and with less sensitivity. The bowel movements are more solid and also occur less frequently—usually only 1 to 2 times per day.

Biting is a habit that should never be allowed to develop. Infants often gum down on hard or cold objects to alleviate the pain associated with teething. When they do this with teeth, and when the hard surface is the bony flesh of another, pain is likely to be inflicted. Parents should be quick to disallow this activity before it becomes a bad habit or as a weapon used to manipulate others or to get their own way.

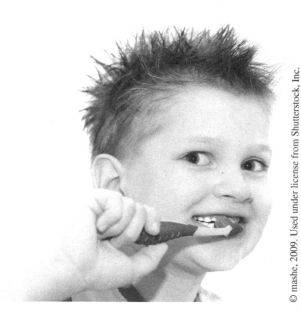

© mashe, 2009. Used under license from Shutterstock, Inc.

Care means more than just hygiene, it also means avoiding foods with high sugar content. One of the most damaging high sugar content foods ingested by infants and toddlers is milk. Milk taken from a cup is swallowed directly and does not harm the enamel of the teeth but milk taken from a nipple tends to accumulate on the backs of the teeth and eat away at the enamel. This is another reason why weaning from the bottle or breast is highly encouraged before age 1.

Many people think that there is no need to take care of primary teeth since they will all be displaced later on, but this is far from the truth. The primary teeth preserve the root beds and the spacing for the secondary teeth so care is definitely indicated.

Growth and Development

Because the heart and lungs increase in size and capacity, the heart and respiratory rates of the toddler decrease from what they were for the infant. The toddler heart rate is approximately 100 to 110 beats per minute and the respiratory rate is 20 to 30 breaths per minute.

The brain of the toddler is continuing to grow and develop. There are now more neural connections that will facilitate cognition and problem-solving ability and the beginning of myelinization that will facilitate gaining body control. Myelinization speeds and refines the transmission of neural messages. This will be essential to learning balance, coordination, and bowel and bladder control.

Other maturational changes include the increased ability of the kidneys to concentrate urine. This makes diaper changes less frequent but bladder control usually is not accomplished until age 3 or 4. The stomach capacity is larger than during infancy allowing the toddler to eat more at one sitting and to eat less frequently. The digestive system is less sensitive to foods so the toddler is now able to eat a greater variety of foods.

Some milestone gross motor achievements for the toddler include learning to climb, jump, skip, run, walk sideways and backwards, stand on tiptoes, and balance on one foot. Some milestone fine motor achievements include the ability to build towers of blocks using up to six blocks, using "fat" pencils or crayons to scribble, copy figures and draw "stick" people, and the ability to feed themselves using small forks and spoons and drinking from a cup.

Nutrition

Obviously, toddlers will continue to gain weight and increase in height but the rate of this growth is substantially less. Toddlers only gain 5 to 6 pounds per year and increase their height by only 4 or 5 inches. With the slowing of growth also comes the slowing of growth requirements. This essentially means that the toddlers have a decreased appetite (as compared to that of the infant). Some parents become unnecessarily concerned about this, but it is perfectly normal.

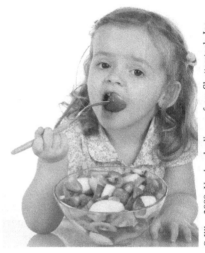

Because toddlers are so busy exploring the world and are so distracted by these ventures, they also do not like to slow down and take time out to eat. Parents and caregivers are encouraged to offer food incentives but not to offer food as a reward. Candy or a trip to McDonald's as a reward for good behavior only sets a precedent that is not easily reversed.

Food Incentives

Food incentives are strategies that will hopefully encourage toddlers to eat. For example, **finger foods** are appealing to toddlers because they can be held in one hand and can be eaten on the run. Examples of finger foods are celery and carrot sticks, peanut butter on crackers, and small pieces of cutup fruits. Toddlers also prefer small portions. Generally speaking, a portion should never exceed the size of the palm of their hands. Toddlers should also never be forced to "clean their plate." They tend to stop eating when they are full. Another food incentive is to serve food in dishes that are compartmentalized. Toddlers do not like to mix foods.

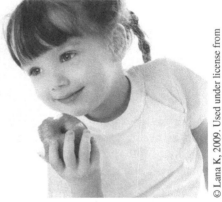

Sometimes toddlers go through phases of **food jags**. They may want peanut butter and jelly every day for a while and then want bologna every day for a few days. This is normal and nothing to worry about as long as the food is nutritious. Wanting cookies and milk every day (without having bologna) would definitely not be encouraged. Of course, the best food incentive for toddlers is role modeling by the parents or caregivers. If parents don't eat vegetables, it is not likely that their children will eat vegetables.

Sleep Requirements

Sleep requirements for the toddler, because of the decreased growth rate, are also less. Most toddlers sleep 10 hours at night plus take a 2-hour nap during the early afternoon. The afternoon nap helps the toddler to recharge for the rest of the day's activities and helps to alleviate or minimize the stress associated with figuring out the world's problems. Most toddlers need bedtime and nap rituals to help them relax sufficiently to sleep restfully. Bedtime rituals are nothing but routines. These routines help the toddler make sense of a very confusing world and to feel more secure in it. An example of a bedtime ritual would be taking a bath, putting on pajamas, brushing teeth, getting into bed, listening to a bedtime story, turning on the night-light, turning off the overhead light, getting a kiss from Mom and Dad with a comment like "sleep tight and I'll see you in the morning," and then seeing the door close. When these routines are not followed in the expected sequence (like when visitors are present or when a babysitter is in charge), the sleep of the toddler can definitely be negatively affected.

© Alicia Shields, 2009. Used under license from Shutterstock, Inc.

Toddlers also tend to cling to familiar objects to help them feel secure. These might be a pacifier, a "security blanket," or a favorite stuffed animal or toy. There is nothing wrong with having these items for security, but it is often a challenge for parents to wean toddlers from them. Generally speaking, it is not socially acceptable to be sucking on a pacifier while sitting in a second grade classroom.

What do you think?

Don't we all STILL have our security blankets? Maybe it's chocolate or a warm bath—but we all retreat to a comfort zone.

Separation Anxiety

Separation anxiety, related to the cognitive ability to comprehend object permanence, can also be a major challenge for parents. Toddlers need to learn to healthily separate from their parents and/or caregivers. Within the home, this is accomplished by encouraging the toddlers to play in rooms that are adjacent to or in view of where the caregivers are, or by having the caregivers check frequently on the toddler. Eventually the toddler learns to trust that they are not alone and can tolerate longer time periods without requiring direct contact with parents. In homes where there are other siblings, or in day care centers when there are other children around, this is accomplished rather quickly. When this is not the case, it is not uncommon for the toddler to create imaginary playmates.

Play

Play is the total order of business for the toddler. Toddlers explore and make sense of the world totally through their play activities. Through play, toddlers obtain lots of physical and mental exercise and they learn to balance and control their bodies. Through play, toddlers improve their muscle coordination and manual dexterity and develop spatial and sensory perceptions.

When several children are playing in the same location, their play can be described as **parallel play**. This means that they are playing side by side without having the need to interact. There may be observation of others and imitation, but very limited communication or interaction of any sort except for maybe defining turf issues relating to what is "mine."

Because of the limited cognition at this stage of development, the toddler's perspective is characterized as being egotistical. Toddlers simply cannot understand the perspective of others. Because of this, toddlers cannot understand why they could or should be expected to share their toys or space and parents should be encouraged not to make this an excessive demand on them. Sharing will become easier during the preschool years.

Play should be spontaneous and creative rather than planned and structured and toys should be without rules. There is nothing wrong with educational toys that help the toddler to sort out shapes and colors and to differentiate sounds and functions but toddlers need to make things work the way they want them to. Toddlers don't really care if irons are intended to take the wrinkles out of clothing. If they can move an iron along the floor like a car or truck, then it is a car or truck. Blocks are great toys for toddlers because they can become whatever the child wants them to be, buildings, cars, telephones, food, and so forth.

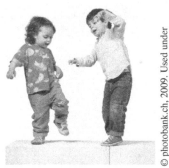
© photobank.ch, 2009. Used under license from Shutterstock, Inc.

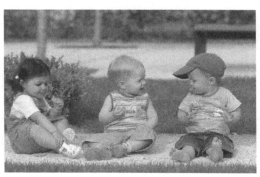
© Vitaliy Hrabar, 2009. Used under license from Shutterstock, Inc.

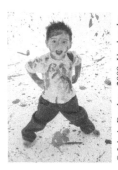
© Jaimie Duplass, 2009. Used under license from Shutterstock, Inc.

The play environment needs to be **childproofed**. This means that medications, sharp objects, sharp edges, toxic chemicals, breakable objects, and anything potentially harmful should be removed. Play time also needs to be supervised. Toddlers are impulsive and move very quickly. Their inquisitive nature and their short attention span can get them into trouble very quickly. They lack judgment about consequences of their actions and toddlers are great imitators. So, if they have seen an adult use a sharp knife to cut up a piece of fruit, they may attempt to do this as well.

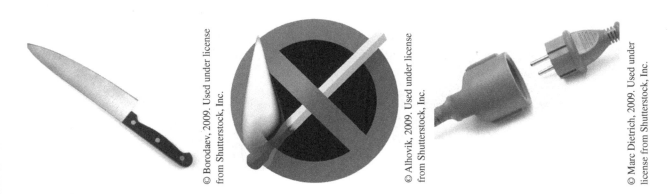
© Borodaev, 2009. Used under license from Shutterstock, Inc.

© Alhovik, 2009. Used under license from Shutterstock, Inc.

© Marc Dietrich, 2009. Used under license from Shutterstock, Inc.

When toddlers are engaged in play, they are totally absorbed. Interrupting or terminating their play too abruptly can be extremely frustrating and may initiate a most unpleasant temper tantrum. Parents and caregivers are advised to help the toddler learn how to bring play time to a gradual closing. Having them put their toys away is a good way to help them recognize that play time is almost over.

Toddlers are all about exploring the world and figuring out how things work. This can get them into serious trouble like when they put a wet finger into a live socket or when they attempt to climb to the top of the

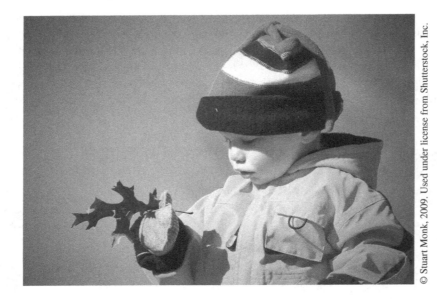

highest cabinet just to see what is inside. Toddlers also like to taste everything not realizing that not all things are intended to be ingested.

Developmental Theories

Autonomy vs. Shame and Doubt (Erik Erikson)

The psychosocial task for toddlers to achieve, according to Erikson (1968) is autonomy. This means that toddlers need to learn how to function at least somewhat independently. Autonomy is achieved through learning self-help skills of everyday living like eating, dressing, toileting, hygiene, and mobility as well as learning some beginning sense of managing frustration and stress. This can be summed up as gaining control over their motor abilities, their sphincters, and their emotions.

Gaining mobility and balance and coordination is relatively easy compared to learning to control sphincters and emotions. With increased practice and experimentation, toddlers learn to walk steadily, run, peddle a tricycle, climb, and skip all by themselves. But it is only with lots of patience and consistency from parents and/or caregivers that toddlers can achieve bowel and bladder control.

Toilet Training

Toilet training also requires that toddlers have sufficient cognition to understand what is expected or desired. If toddlers do not have any clue about why they are sitting on a potty chair or if they do not receive praise from their parents for fulfilling their wishes or desires, then nothing will be accomplished.

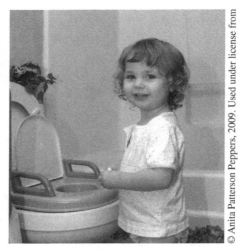

Toilet training involves helping toddlers to gain bowel and bladder control. Bowel training is easier than bladder control because bowel movements occur less frequently. Bowel training cannot occur until or unless there is myelinization of the nerves in the spinal tract. This usually does not occur until around age 2.

Once myelinization has occurred, toddlers become aware of the sensation of fullness and the need to defecate. Sometimes, when toddlers first become aware of this sensation, they may become red in the face or retreat to a corner and squat. This is a telltale sign that parents should recognize and then escort the child to a potty chair.

This sensation must be felt or there cannot be toilet training. Prior to this innervation, parents who are lucky enough to "catch" stool in a potty chair are training themselves rather than their toddlers. Toddlers need to be helped to recognize that this sensation is a cue to use the bathroom. Learning to respond to this sensation in a timely manner is a major accomplishment.

Learning to Control Emotions

Another major challenge in helping toddlers achieve autonomy is related to emotions. Toddlerhood is often referred to as "the terrible 2's" because toddlers are notorious for saying "NO" and for throwing temper tantrums.

Toddlers learn the word *no* from their parents. Because toddlers are so inquisitive and impulsive, they do tend to do things that they shouldn't. When this occurs, parents react with a loud and resounding "no." So, when parents make demands on the toddler that the toddler doesn't want, they use this same weapon. To minimize this occurrence, parents and caregivers are encouraged to use distraction and/or removal from the source of less than desirable activities rather than to say no.

Did you know?

Did you know that most day care center employees are educated NOT to use the word "no"? In these settings, it is rare to hear "no" from the children.

Parents are also encouraged to give the toddler alternative choices rather than to ask them or tell them to do one thing. For example, asking a toddler if they prefer peanut butter or bologna is more likely to get a positive response than to ask if they want peanut butter. This latter question might very likely get a "no" response, while the alternative strategy helps the toddler to feel that they are in charge.

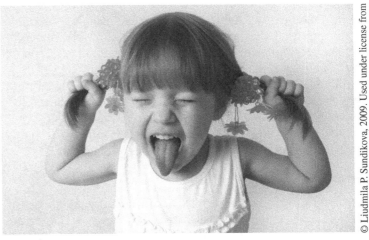

© Liudmila P. Sundikova, 2009. Used under license from Shutterstock, Inc.

Temper tantrums are usually evidences of frustration. Because needs were met so promptly and consistently during infancy, it is a big shock to toddlers to learn that they will not always get everything they want or when they want it. Learning delayed gratification is extremely frustrating for toddlers and when they don't know what else to do, they just cry or scream or kick their feet or roll around on the floor.

If toddlers get what they want when they throw these temper tantrums, they tend to repeat the performance. But temper tantrums tend to be self-limiting when they are cautiously ignored. When toddlers learn that their tantrums are not accomplishing anything, they tend to stop.

Autonomy is achieved when toddlers learn to control their bodies, their sphincters, and their emotions without feeling embarrassed or exposed or unsure. When parents and caregivers put too much pressure on the toddler to achieve these tasks or when the toddlers are criticized for not making progress as quickly as desired by the parents, it is likely that shame and doubt will occur.

Preoperational and Preconceptual Cognition and Problem Solving (Piaget)

According to Piaget (1950), cognition and problem solving is transitioning from sensorimotor to preoperational and preconceptual thinking. Toddlers still engage in some trial-and-error experimentation (trying to manipulate a large cookie into milk that is in a glass with a small diameter) but now there is some beginning of internal representation (thinking about it first) involved in problem solving. This means that, with the added assets of memory and language, toddlers can begin to figure things out without necessarily physically manipulating them. In the example above, they may conclude that the cookie needs to be broken in half.

This level of cognition, according to Piaget, is parataxic, meaning that it is simply what it is; that is, hot is hot, and cold is cold. There is essentially no cause and effect and no wholeness. For example regarding cause and effect, toddlers are unable to comprehend consequences. Telling them that something may harm them means nothing to them. That is why parents need to so carefully supervise toddler activity and to childproof the environment. This is also why parents are so tempted to say "no" to so many activities. Parataxic cognition also involves transductive reasoning, meaning that black is black and white is white and there are no broad categories or subcategories. For example, a rose is a rose and nothing more. It is not a flower or a plant; it is only a rose.

The thinking of a toddler is also egocentric. This means that toddlers are truly unable to understand the perspective of others. This means that their thinking is self-absorbed but not in an intentional, selfish way as this term implies for adults. Toddlers really cannot understand why others don't see things the way they do.

Language

Toddlers do not have an extensive vocabulary and are usually not very verbal in their interactions. The language of a toddler is syncretic and telegraphic, meaning that one or two words mean more. An example of this is "milk" means "I want a cup of milk" and "go outside" means "I want to go outside and play." The language of the toddler is sometimes described as being autistic, meaning that it has meaning only to the child. Nonetheless, language should be encouraged.

Allowing a toddler to grunt and point without making a verbal request is too often tolerated by parents and caregivers. It would be better to tell the child to call whatever they want by name. For example, "If you want a glass of milk, say 'I want milk.'" Similarly, when toddlers refer to objects incorrectly, it is advised to repeat the word correctly and have them repeat it. This minimizes "baby talk" and helps the toddler to build a correct and extensive vocabulary.

Morality

According to Kohlberg's (1969) theory of morality, toddlers are at the Punishment and Obedience Stage. In this stage, toddlers will do what they can get away with. For example, a toddler may not pull the dog's tail while the parents are in the room because they know that the parents will tell them "no," or swat their hands or move them away from the dog. But, when the parents are not in the room, there is absolutely no reason why they could not or should not do this.

Because of this limited level of thinking and perspective, it is critical that punishments for unacceptable behavior be appropriate to the offense. Distraction works to stop the undesirable activity but does not necessarily help the toddler to know that this activity is not to be repeated. That is why the parent's tone of voice while saying "no" is so often invoked. Time-out only works if the child understands that what they were doing is wrong. When they know that they will be required to endure this isolation if they get caught, it may be incentive enough for them not to do it. Time-outs should never be longer in minutes than the age of the child. Time-out for a 2-year-old should never exceed 2 minutes.

Parenting

Parenting of a toddler requires lots of skills. Parents need to know the limitations of thinking during toddlerhood so they will have realistic expectations. Parents need to consistently praise and reinforce positive behaviors, offer alternative choices, avoid negativism and criticism, provide safe areas for play, and avoid overprotection and/or isolation.

As in all ages, motor vehicle accidents are the number one cause of accidental death for toddlers. Other accidents from falls, burns, poisoning, and drowning are also possible but preventable with adequate supervision by parents and caregivers.

Common Illnesses

Otitis media is the most common toddler illness but, if recognized early, can be successfully treated with antibiotics. Other problems occurring during this age are respiratory problems such as croup, bronchitis, asthma, and pneumonia. Chronic conditions, such as cerebral palsy and muscular dystrophy, even though present from birth, may become apparent during this stage of development because of the expected gross motor milestone achievements. During this stage, kidney syndromes may also become apparent.

Hospitalization is traumatic at any age but is particularly traumatic for toddlers. Toddlers perceive hospitalization as punishment and isolation. This results in separation anxiety that may cause problems for many years to come. The reaction to this separation might be protest (evident by persistent crying), despair (evident by withdrawal, passive, regressive behaviors), or denial (evident in superficial, non-emotional responses). Parents are encouraged to stay with toddlers during necessary hospitalizations and are also encouraged to try to maintain daily routines as much as possible.

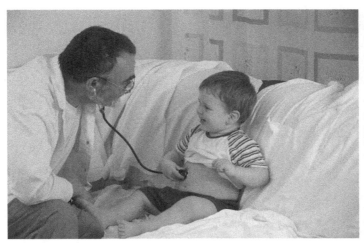

© Viktor Pryymachuk, 2009. Used under license from Shutterstock, Inc.

Summary

Toddlerhood is a very busy time. Toddlers are constantly exploring and discovering and re-defining their world. It is a trying time for many parents and caregivers especially relating to toilet training and temper tantrums, but it is a delightful time to see this little person emerge into their own unique identity.

References

Erikson, E. H. (1968). *Childhood and society* (35th anniversary ed.). New York: Norton.

Kohlberg, L. (1981). *The philosophy of moral development: Vol. 1.* San Francisco: Harper & Row.

Piaget, J. (1950). *The psychology of intelligence.* London: Routledge and Kegan Paul.

Reflection

In the space below, recall and describe an encounter you may have had with a toddler and explain if this confirms or denies the theory as related in this chapter.

Assignment

Complete this form with essential data for a Toddler

Growth and Development Guide for Toddler

	Physical Traits	Physical Abilities	Psychosocial Task (Erikson)	Evidence of How Achieved	Evidence of Non-Achievement	Cognitive Ability (Piaget)	Evidence of Achievement	Moral Capability (Kohlberg)	Evidence of Achievement
Toddler (1–3 years)									

Study Guide for Toddler
(1–3 Years)

1. Describe the toddler appearance as opposed to that of an infant: head, chest, limbs.

2. Describe the organ maturation (and implications) of toddlers as compared to infants.

3. Differentiate the nutritional and sleep requirements for toddlers compared to that for infants.

4. Describe the play of a toddler: type of play and what is gained in this experience.

5. Explain what self-care independence means and give examples.

6. Identify the pre-requirements that are essential PRIOR to beginning toilet training.

7. Identify and give examples of how a toddler learns body control (gross motor and fine motor skills).

8. What is the meaning of 'delayed gratification' and how is this learned by the toddler?

9. Give an example of Trial and Error cognition.

10. Explain how and why the behavior of a toddler is governed by a 'punishment vs. obedience' perspective.

Name: _____

Review

1. Why do toddlers establish ritualistic behavior patterns?

    a. to reestablish their sense of identity
    b. to learn new activities
    c. to manipulate and control adults in their environment
    d. to feel secure among the inconsistencies of their world

2. Which of the following would be considered uncharacteristic of toddler behavior?

    a. can readily accept delay and frustration
    b. develops motor skills before language and problem-solving skills
    c. is driven by curiosity to explore surroundings
    d. develops socialization and beginning problem solving ability through play

3. What is characteristic of a 'food jag'?

    a. refusing to eat
    b. crying every time one is made to sit down to eat
    c. wanting the same food over and over again
    d. playing with food more than eating it

4. Which of the following is the best technique to avoid hearing 'NO' from a toddler?

    a. phrase requests as alternatives rather than in yes or no format
    b. offer incentives in order to get them to do what you want
    c. make them sit in 'time out' every time they say 'no'
    d. don't make any requests of the toddler

G&D: TODDLER

• TODDLER -- age 1-3
Physical Characteristics
Chest now a bit larger than head

© photobank.ch, 2009

Short legs; protruding abdomen, wide stance and waddled walk

Thickening of skin: < vulnerable to rashes / injury

Images used under license from Shutterstock, Inc.

G&D: TODDLER

TODDLER TEETH
16 Primary teeth
the more to chew with;
the more to bite with

© mashe, 2009

Need oral hygiene as soon as teeth erupt
to sustain health of gums and nerves
(roots) for secondary teeth
& to sustain spacing for Secondary
teeth

Images used under license from Shutterstock, Inc.

HR Babies 120-160
Toddlers-

G&D: TODDLER

TODDLER
Heart and Lung capacity larger so now able to sustain higher energy level
Heart Rate decreases to 100-110 beats/minute;
Respiratory rate decreases to 20-30 breaths/minute

Kidneys more mature and developed so now able to increase concentration which means less frequent urinations and/or diaper changes

Bowel Movement 2-3 hrs
- Potty Trained

G&D: TODDLER

TODDLER BRAIN
approximating full anatomical size but still
undergoing lots of development inside

Axons/dendrites/synapses = networking
and connections
Myelinization = speed of neural
transmission and speed of sensory reception

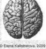

© Elena Kalistratova, 2009

Images used under license from Shutterstock, Inc.

Fael sensation to urinate.

G&D: TODDLER

Stomach capacity larger than during infancy
now able to eat more at one sitting and to eat less
frequently

Digestive system less sensitive
now able to eat greater variety of foods

Much slower growth rate than during infancy
Weight gain: 5-6 pounds/year
Height increase: 4-5 inches/year

G&D: TODDLER

• TODDLER NUTRITION
  • Toddlers do NOT like to take time out to eat
    Too busy exploring and conquering the world

  • But they don't need as many calories as
    during infancy because their growth is
    now at a slower pace

  • And they need to learn to use utensils: forks and spoons

© Ilike, 2009

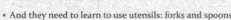

Images used under license from Shutterstock, Inc.

Do Not like for food to mix
Food Jags- onething for a bit
while

G&D: TODDLER

- Food Incentives for Toddlers:
  - Give advance warning when interrupting play time
  - Offer 'Finger foods'
  - Small servings (palm of hand) in compartmentalized dishes
  - Tolerance of 'food jags'
  - Avoidance of using food as reward
  - Avoidance of requirement to 'clean plate'
  - Importance of Role Modeling

© Lana K, 2009

Images used under license from Shutterstock, Inc.

Develop Healthy Eating Habits

G&D: TODDLER

- SLEEP REQUIREMENTS FOR TODDLERS
  - Requirement less related to slower growth rate
    - 10 hours/night plus 1-2 hr nap during day
  - Bedtime rituals
    - Sequence of activities
    - Consistency of time and routine = security
    - Security blankets okay but should be weaned before entry into school

Images used under license from Shutterstock, Inc.

G&D: TODDLER

- Separation Anxiety
  - Related to awareness of
  - Object Permanence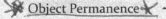
    Need to encourage toddlers to play in rooms that are adjacent to or in view of where the caregivers are, or by having the caregivers check frequently on the toddler.
  - Difficult time for parents leaving child with baby-sitter

9 mnth of age

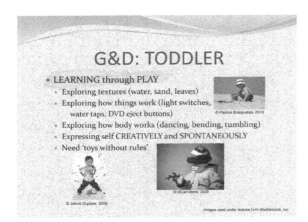

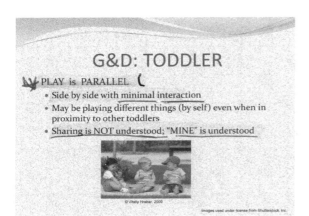

G&D: TODDLER

- PLAY should be SAFE
  - Childproofed
    Removal of objects that may cause harm or injury

    Play equipment and/or toys with soft rounded edges
    Play environment with soft surface (sand or grass)
  - SUPERVISED: Toddlers are impulsive and FAST!!!

Images used under license from Shutterstock, Inc.

G&D: TODDLER

- Developmental Theories
- Erik Erikson: Autonomy vs. Shame and Doubt
  - Gaining control of body (Gross Motor Skills)
    - Balance, running (stopping ???) climbing, pedaling
    - Body control, muscle tone and coordination, and development of spatial and sensory perceptions

© anetta, 2009

Images used under license from Shutterstock, Inc.

G&D: TODDLER

- Developmental Theories
- Erik Erikson: Autonomy vs. Shame and Doubt
  - Gaining control of body (Fine Motor Skills)
    - building blocks;
    - using 'fat' crayons
    - learning manual dexterity

© Dagmara Ponikewska, 2009

Images used under license from Shutterstock, Inc.

G&D: TODDLER

- PSYCHOSOCIAL TASK (Erikson) -- AUTONOMY
  - Doing it myself!
    - Gaining control over body and activities of daily living
      - Dressing: choices
      - Eating: preferences
      - Playing: selection and timing

Images used under license from Shutterstock, Inc.

Autonomy – "I am in control of my own world, I can DO IT"
└ Want to be independent
w/ confidence
Shame & Doubt – Potty Training

G&D: TODDLER

Toileting:

Bowel before bladder but neither until/unless

a. myelizination of spinal cord

b. regularity

c. understanding of expectations

Images used under license from Shutterstock, Inc.

G&D: TODDLER

- PSYCHOSOCIAL TASK (Erikson) -- AUTONOMY
  Gaining control over Emotions!

Temper Tantrums – frustration (self-limiting)

Saying "NO"

Learning delayed gratification

Images used under license from Shutterstock, Inc.

Set guidelines instead of saying NO

b/c have no coping mechanisms.

G&D: TODDLER

- COGNITION (Piaget)
  - Problem solving transition from sensorimotor to
    - Pre-Operational (Internal Representation)
      - Memory
      - Language
    - Egotistic – do not understand perspective of others
    - Parataxic – it is what it is (hot is hot; cold is cold)
      do not understand cause & effect and/or consequences
    - Centered – describe objects by single trait or function –
      'a ball is round' or 'a ball bounces' (not both)
    - Transductive – general to general
      all green things with leaves are trees, not bushes or plants or flowers

G&D: TODDLER

* LANGUAGE
  * Syncretic – one word phrase means whole sentence
    * "outside" = I want to go outside
      Progesses to two word phrases like "go outside"
      then to full sentences by age 4
  * Facilitated by modeling (no baby talk) by parents

  * Facilitated by asking toddler to call people and objects
    by name rather than pointing and grunting

  * Facilitated by parents reading to toddler

G&D: TODDLER

* **MORALITY**
  (dependent upon cognitive limitations)

* Toddlers are egotistic (are not capable of understanding
  perspective of others)
* Without understanding cause & effect, a toddler act as he
  pleases until stopped or punished
  * Time out (one minute for each year of age)
  * Distraction
  * Stern voice with "NO" *w/ safety*

Serves as a deterrent to some actions but parents must
consistently enforce expectations and must constantly
SUPERVISE

G&D: TODDLER

* Punishment and Obedience (Kohlberg)

  = I am not doing this because it is right or
  good;

  = I am only doing this because I will be in
  trouble if I don't

  = I will only do this while you are watching;
  don't expect me to do this all the time

G&D: TODDLER

PARENTING of TODDLERS

- Requires Patience and Consistency while attempting to
  - re-inforce positive behaviors,
  - offer alternative choices,
  - avoid negativism and criticism,
  - provide safe areas for play, and
  - avoid overprotection and/or isolation

and SUPERVISE!

G&D: TODDLER

- Common Toddler Injuries
  - MVA, falls, burns, poisonings, drownings

© Viktor Pryymachuk, 2009

- Common Toddler Illnesses
  - Otitis Media, croup, bronchitis, asthma, pneumonia and renal conditions *Ear Infection*

- Hospitalization during toddlerhood is especially traumatic → Protest, Despair, Denial
  - From Separation Anxiety – Moms need to stay with toddlers
  - And often causing Regression (loss of autonomy)

Images used under license from Shutterstock, Inc.

Preschool (3–5 Years)

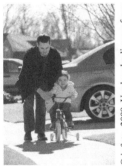

© iofoto, 2009. Used under license from Shutterstock, Inc.

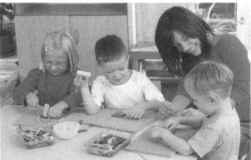

© matka_Wariatka, 2009. Used under license from Shutterstock, Inc.

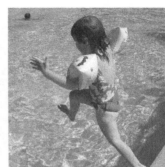

© Oxana Prokofyeva, 2009. Used under license from Shutterstock, Inc.

Objectives

Upon completion of this chapter, the reader should be able to:

1. Compare and contrast the physical characteristics, growth rate, and nutritional needs of the preschooler with those of the infant and toddler.
2. Describe the psychosocial task of initiative as theorized by Erikson to be evidenced in the preschool years.
3. Describe the cognitive capabilities of preschoolers as theorized by Piaget.
4. Compare and contrast the play characteristics of a preschooler as compared to that of a toddler.
5. Describe positive parenting practices for preschoolers.

Key Terms

Cause and Effect: the cognitive ability to recognize that A leads to B, that is, that certain actions will result in predictable consequences

Centering: the cognitive limitation of focusing on only one aspect of a situation or one feature of an object at a time without recognizing that multiple characteristics exist

Cooperative play: a form of play activity that demands assuming of roles, organization, sequencing, and interaction with others for an intended outcome

Regression: reverting to behaviors and actions of a younger person in order to attract the attention that was received before reaching the current level of maturation

Reversibility: a cognitive ability that recognizes that matter, even in different forms, remains the same matter

Sibling rivalry: jealousy and resentment of perceived infringement of space, time, and affection from parents, usually from an older sibling towards a younger one, which may result in attempts to regain priority status

Transductive logic: a cognitive limitation that assumes that similar objects are known by the same term, that is, a dog is a dog without recognizing the variations in breed

Characteristics of the Preschooler

The preschool years are exciting years. The preschooler is no longer dependent upon their caregivers for basic activities of daily living. They can dress and feed themselves and can use the bathroom facilities without assistance. They can express their needs in words and sentences and can tell stories in proper sequence. They can play independently and they can play interactively without an egotistic perspective. Preschoolers have greater control of their fine muscles and so can draw and color pictures, can print their name, and can even tie their shoes. This is the beginning of knowing who and what they are and what they want to do or be.

The preschooler is more proportional in physique. Their chest is now larger than the head, and their legs have grown longer so they now look more like a small adult. The preschooler now only grows approximately 2½ to 3 inches per year and gains less than 5 pounds per year. Because of this slower growth rate, the nutritional requirements are limited to 1200 to 1600 calories per day. They still require approximately 9 to 11 hours of sleep per night but most preschoolers, by age 5, will no longer require a nap.

The preschooler has a full set of primary teeth (28) and can readily learn how to brush and floss. It is important for parents to teach them to take care of their teeth because these teeth hold space and healthy tissue for the secondary teeth that will follow. Decay in primary teeth establishes an unhealthy environment for the secondary teeth. So just because these teeth are replaced is not a reason to ignore dental hygiene. And it is extremely important for preschoolers to see a dentist at least twice a year for checkups.

Teeth can also be used as a weapon but biting is more common in the toddler than during the preschool stage. Biting is a form of aggression as a means to get what they want and must be curtailed at the first occurrence.

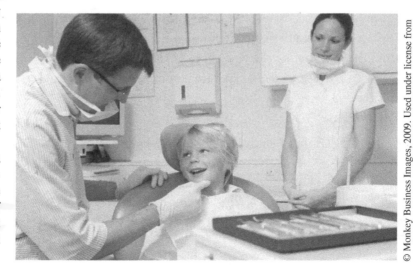

© Monkey Business Images, 2009. Used under license from Shutterstock, Inc.

Safety Considerations

Safety is a major concern during the preschool years. Even though preschoolers are able to dress and feed and toilet themselves, they do not have the judgment to always make the best choices. Preschoolers are also strongly inclined to imitate adults and this can make for a very dangerous situation. Preschoolers are fasci-nated by adult gadgets such as cigarette lighters and matches and they are even more fascinated by the fire that is pro-duced by these items. A major contrib-utor to fires in homes is the unfortunate occurrence of preschoolers playing with matches.

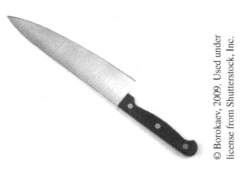
© Mudassar Ahmed Dar, 2009. Used under license from Shutterstock, Inc.

Enforcing the need to use car safety seats and seat belts is critical. Automo-bile accidents are the number one cause of accidental death in all ages, and for preschoolers, this is no exception.

Because preschoolers are now more coordinated in their physical capabili-ties, they often attempt activities that are beyond their ability. Preschoolers need supervision and vigilance when engag-ing in swimming and other outdoor play activities. Indoors, preschoolers also need supervision because they may attempt to perform tasks usually only safely done by adults, such as using a sharp knife or turning on the stove or using toxic cleaning supplies. Medications are also a concern because, when and if the pre-schooler has witnessed parents taking these med-ications, they may assume that they could and should do the same.

© Borokaev, 2009. Used under license from Shutterstock, Inc.

Preschoolers are particularly vulnerable to the kindness and lure of predators. Stranger safety must be instilled at a very early age. This means that preschoolers need to know that not all indi-viduals have their best intentions at heart. Pre-schoolers need to know to whom they can speak and respond and where this is appropriate. Preschoolers also need to learn that "secrets" are never to be kept from parents. Preschoolers also need to learn how to seek help and assistance when needed. They need to know their name, address, and phone number so that in the event that they do become separated from their parents, they can be found.

Play Characteristics

The play time of preschoolers is very different from that of a toddler. Whereas the toddler, with a limited egotis-tic perspective, plays parallel to others but not with them, the preschooler almost always wants interaction. The play of preschoolers is very orchestrated, that is, is planned and structured with specific roles and anticipated outcomes. Much of this play is imitative play, such as pretending to be mother and father, teacher and student,

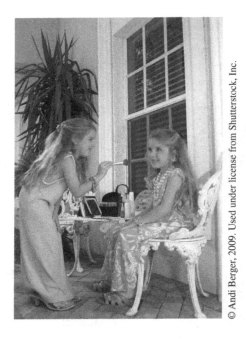

bus driver and rider, superman and victim, doctor and patient, policeman and bad guy, and so on. These play sessions demand that each participant know and carry out their role according to the "rules". In these play sessions, preschoolers learn leader and follower roles, sharing, healthy competition, imagination, creativity, and initiative.

Preschoolers also engage in creative play in activities such as drawing, cutting, pasting, coloring, and painting. It is important to allow the creativity and spontaneity of preschoolers to emerge during these sessions rather than prescribe a certain way to draw this or that. Copying is not the same as drawing. It is equally important to praise their creations. Asking "what in the world is this?" is NOT a positive reaction. Saying, "tell me all about what you drew" is a much better comment.

Music is also a wonderful means of play for preschoolers. They do not need to know how to read music to make sounds and to keep rhythm, and they love to do this. Dancing is also a great way for preschoolers to express their individuality as well as their coordination and sense of rhythm.

Good to know:

Preschoolers thrive on attention and praise from adults. This encourages them to be spontaneous and initiate additional projects that are likely to be praised.
A common acknowledgment of their accomplishments is seen when parents post the drawings of their preschooler on the wall or refrigerator.

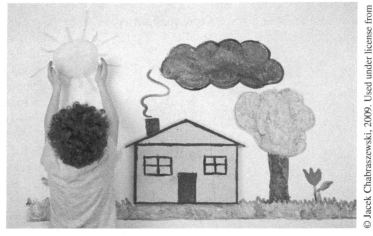

Developmental Theories

Initiative vs. Guilt (Erik Erikson)

The psychosocial developmental task for preschoolers, according to Erikson (1968), is initiative. The opposing resulting trait is guilt. That is, preschoolers learn to spontaneously take initiative in their actions when encouraged and praised. When preschoolers receive ridicule and excessive restrictions, they may develop a tendency to be hesitant about action and feel guilty about doing anything unless directed to do so. The world is full of individuals who fear action because of fear of consequences. Could this be evidence that they were not successful in accomplishing the task of initiative during their preschool years?

With initiative comes increased dependability, cooperation, assertiveness, and organization. These are all good outcomes. With guilt comes assuming responsibility for actions that were not intended, like spilling milk when trying to pour it into a bowl of cereal, like breaking a picture frame while trying to help Mom with dusting, like dropping and losing a nail or screw while trying to help Dad mount a painting on the wall. Guilt results when parents, impatient with results, yell at or punish children for accidents. Positive parenting demands recognizing the intent of the action rather than the end result. For example, even though the preschooler picked the prize rose from your rose garden, it is important to recognize that this was done to show you how much they love you.

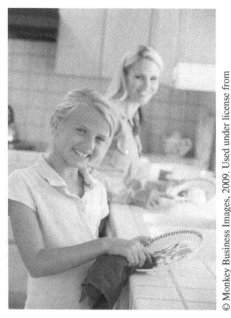

© Monkey Business Images, 2009. Used under license from Shutterstock, Inc.

Preschoolers are full of energy and need to be allowed to express it. They thrive on adult approval and so can be encouraged to maximize their potential. For example, telling them that they are a big boy or girl who can help Mom or Dad may result in their desire to make their bed, clean their room, put away toys, set the table, take out the trash, and so on. This is their choice and their desire to please. It is NOT an order. Watching them beam with pride when Mom or Dad praises them for being so helpful is a joy beyond measure. This is simply a matter of encouragement and should never become bribery with money or candy or outings. If bribery becomes the standard, children will never do anything unless there is some type of reward involved.

Did you know?

Did you know that because preschoolers are so eager to please adults, this is a prime time to engage them in household responsibilities? The activities make them feel grown up and important and it also teaches them family accountability.

Of course, even though parents don't want to discourage spontaneous actions of preschoolers, there are ways to guide the choices that are made. For example, show the preschooler that some flowers are okay to be picked and others that are not. Parents can also encourage the preschooler to ask for assistance when needed. This, of course, means that parents must be willing to assist when asked. Deferring this opportunity may result in the preschooler's failed attempt and negative results. For example, parents may encourage the preschooler to ask them to pour the milk from the large container into a small measuring cup so that the preschooler can then independently pour the milk on the cereal. This way, initiative is accomplished and both parent and child can feel good about themselves and the situation.

There is a phenomenon that frequently occurs during the preschool years known as the Oedipal Complex. This term comes from Freud's (1961) psychoanalytic theory that is essentially sexually based. The term comes from Greek mythology about the love affair between a mother and son, even though they were unaware of their kinship. According to Freud, during the preschool period, girls tend to compete with their mothers for the love and affection of their fathers and boys compete with their fathers for the love and affection of their mothers. This may be seen in the girl's' attempts to dress, wear makeup, and walk and talk like their mother. Boys similarly may take on the characteristics of their fathers. More recent theories indicate that this is mostly imitation and gender identity rather anything with sexual overtones.

Preoperational Cognition (Piaget)

According to Piaget (1950), the cognitive ability of the preschooler involves some trial-and-error strategies but is now more intuitive. The preschooler has sufficient memory that allows them to figure out solutions in their mind rather than by necessarily having to physically manipulate objects. A classic example of this is learning that breaking a cookie in half, so that it fits into a cup or glass of milk, will make dunking more efficient. A toddler might very well try to force the whole cookie into the cup.

There are still lots of limitations in the thinking of a preschooler though. They tend to **center** on situations, that is, they can only perceive one aspect at a time. For example, they can understand that they are a girl, but they may not be able to simultaneously perceive that they are also a daughter, a sister, a niece, or a granddaughter. They may know that a ball is round or that its color is red, but they cannot put it all together to know that this red, round ball can bounce, roll, and be thrown and kicked. Preschoolers can usually only think of one perspective at a time.

Another cognitive limitation, closely associated with centering, is known as **transductive logic**. This simply means that preschoolers think of objects in terms of specific to specific rather than from general to specific. In the thinking of a preschooler, a rose is a rose and anything that resembles a rose is a rose. A rose is therefore not a flower in the mind of a preschooler and a dog is a dog without differentiating the many breeds and sizes.

Preschoolers also think in absolutes. For example, they may think that all girls have long hair and all boys have short hair. So, if they encounter a girl with short hair, they may well assume that this is a boy. Similarly they may think of their parent's occupation as the only occupation, that is, someone else's parents aren't really going to work if they go to another site.

Preschoolers are not yet capable of understanding **reversibility**. Reversibility means that individuals are able to recognize that objects in one form can be changed and then returned to its original state. For example, water can become ice and then become water again. Another example is that play dough can be shaped into a form and then wadded back into a ball of nothing but dough. According to a preschooler, it is either water or ice, not the same matter; it is either dough or a donkey, not the same matter. The cognitive ability to recognize the reversibility of objects becomes apparent in the school-age years.

Preschoolers also have limited ability relating to **cause and effect**. They understand that something is hot but they cannot understand the implications of becoming burned. They understand that they should not go into the street, but they cannot understand the implications of being hit by a car. They know that they may not do certain things because doing so may get them in trouble but not necessarily because they understand the rationale. Learning that certain behaviors or activities may hurt them is usually all that can be hoped for when trying to explain to preschoolers about potential dangers.

Instilling a certain degree of fear and caution related to some actions is a good thing. But when excessive, preschoolers could develop unwarranted fears. For example, recognizing that "dogs may bite" is okay as long as the preschoolers don't fear this so much that they run scared every time they encounter a dog. Knowing that doors should be locked to prevent unwanted intruders may cause a preschooler to fantasize that someone is always "out there" and ready to break in at any given moment. These unwarranted fears often are the source of nightmares, sleepwalking, and bedwetting. It is not always easy for parents to know how much fear and how much encouragement should be instilled. A general rule of thumb, as always, is moderation.

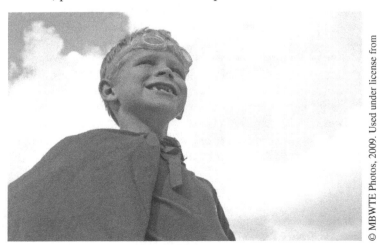

© MBWTE Photos, 2009. Used under license from Shutterstock, Inc.

Preschoolers are also known for their frequent **intermingling of fantasy with reality**. They are fascinated with superheroes and saving the world but this does not mean that when superman falls off the swing that he won't cry and run to Mom for comfort. Preschoolers may believe that there is a little elf inside their ears that is working hard to help them to hear or that a giant rabbit will bring them a basket of goodies at Easter. This fantasy world is all part of their imagination and creativity.

It is this intermingling of fantasy with reality that also contributes to some preschoolers creating "imaginary friends." This is more common in preschoolers who are cared for in homes without other siblings or where they are lacking the opportunity for re-al-life intermingling with other children.

Language

Language becomes explosive during the preschool years. The 300-word vocabulary of a toddler that was limited to nouns and simple verbs expands dramatically during the preschool years. Preschoolers now have a vocabulary of more than 3000 words and can form sentences, use correct tense, and tell stories in sequence. They love to recall events and tell everything that happened. It is not uncommon for them to say "and then…" over and over. They are also able to define words but this is usually in terms of function (remember the limitation of centering). For example, when asked "what is a lake?" they would probably say it is where boats go up and down rather than a body of water.

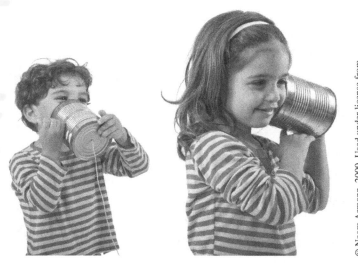

© Noam Armonn, 2009. Used under license from Shutterstock, Inc.

It is often debated about the advantages of having babies and young children reared in a household in which two languages are spoken. Evidence clearly favors this practice when possible. Exposure to a second language, even though starting during in-fancy, becomes fruitful beyond belief during the preschool period. It is truly remarkable how preschoolers are able to use the correct words in the correct language and in the correct tense without too much prompting.

Did you know?

Did you know that it is not until the pre-school age that children are able to dif-ferentiate prepositions like "behind," "in front of," "on top of," "next to"? These important words in our language facilitate specific directional requests.

Morality: Instrumental Purpose and Exchange (Kohlberg)

The moral perspective of a preschooler, according to Kohlberg (1969), is Instrumental Purpose and Exchange. This just simply means "what am I going to get in return?" For the most part, preschoolers strive to get praise and encouragement and this IS their return. They do not need money or gifts; they want the pride and pleasure that is evident in their parents' smiles and words.

Preschoolers still decide about some actions based on "fear and punishment," but are now capable of choosing actions and determining whether or not these actions will bring pleasure to Mom and Dad or not. This is a definite progression in moral thinking and is related to their increased cognitive ability to understand the perspective of others. They are no longer limited to an egotistical perspective. Instrumental Purpose and Exchange also allows preschoolers to comfort others when hurt, to share toys, and to take turns.

A challenge to parents during the preschool period is the situation of **sibling rivalry**. This is jealousy and resentment of perceived infringement of space, time, and affection from parents, usually from an older sibling towards a younger one, which may result in attempts to regain priority status. Preschoolers, sensing that they are less important or less loved than the younger sibling, may regress to activities exhibited in the younger sibling. This may take the form of drinking from a nippled bottle or wetting their pants. Another result might be aggression, which may cause them to inflict some physical harm to the younger sibling. Parents need to recognize this possibility and make sure that the older sibling feels equally prized and treasured. Having big girl or big boy time for reading a story or playing, and creating "just us" situations, goes a long way to reassure the preschooler that they are still a priority.

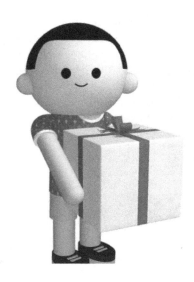 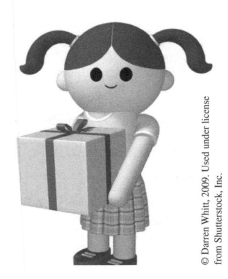

© Darren Whitt, 2009. Used under license from Shutterstock, Inc.

Health Maintenance

Preschoolers need to have regular checkups with their pediatricians in order to receive the required vaccines and to identify, as early as possible, any problems that may occur either physically or developmentally. Unfortunately, some preschoolers develop infections, injuries, or malignancies that require medicinal or surgical intervention. Hospitalization can be especially traumatic to a child teeming with energy and initiative. Hospitalization tends to make the preschooler feel isolated and may result in regression or aggression. To minimize these effects and the stress of the situation, parents are encouraged to stay with the child during these necessary hospital stays and to try to make their daily routines as normal as possible.

Parents should also be alert to any indication that their preschooler may have a vision or hearing deficit. Without optimal hearing and vision, the child may have limited success in school or in social interactions. Hearing and vision deficits can usually be compensated for and accommodated with the aid of eyeglasses and hearing aids.

Summary

Parenting of preschoolers demands lots and lots of vigilance, lots and lots of praise, lots and lots of encouragement, answering whys with simple and direct responses, explaining simple cause-and-effect perspectives, and constantly reinforcing positive behaviors. This is not an easy task but can be accomplished with patience and nurturing.

Parents also need to prevent injury to preschoolers. This is accomplished best by supervision. Without supervision, preschoolers, with their vivid imagination and propensity for imitation, may engage themselves in activities that could result in serious injury. As with toddlers, the most common injuries of preschoolers include automobile accidents, burns, drownings, and falls.

References

Erikson, E. H. (1968). *Childhood and society* (35th anniversary ed.). New York: Norton.

Freud, S. (1961). The resistances to psycho-analysis. *In The Standard Edition of the Complete Psychological Works of Sigmund Freud, Volume XIX* (1923–1925): The Ego and the Id and other works (pp. 211–224).

Kohlberg, L. (1981). *The philosophy of moral development: Vol. 1.* San Francisco: Harper & Row.

Piaget, J. (1950). *The psychology of intelligence.* London: Routledge and Kegan Paul.

Reflection

In the space below, recall how you felt as a young child when your mother or father bragged about you to someone else. Describe this occasion.

If you can't recall something about yourself, think about something you witnessed in a preschool child that evidenced initiative, or demonstrated guilt and describe this event.

Assignment

Complete this form with essential data for Preschool

Growth and Development Guide for Preschool

	Physical Traits	Physical Abilities	Psychosocial Task (Erikson)	Evidence of How Achieved	Evidence of Non-Achievement	Cognitive Ability (Piaget)	Evidence of Achievement	Moral Capability (Kohlberg)	Evidence of Achievement
Preschool (3–5 years)									

Name: _____

Study Guide for
Preschool (3–5 Years)

1. Compare and contrast the appearance of a preschooler to a toddler.

2. Give two examples of how a preschooler might demonstrate initiative.

3. Give two examples of how a preschooler might demonstrate guilt.

4. Describe what is meant by intuitive thought and give at least one example of this.

5. Describe what is meant by a preschooler's 'language explosion'.

6. Compare and contrast the play of a preschooler to that of a toddler.

7. Describe what is meant by the 'Oedipal Complex' as sometimes observed in a preschooler.

8. Relate a preschooler's limitation in understanding cause and effect to the possibility of unwarranted fears.

9. Describe what is meant by 'Instrumental Purpose and Exchange' and relate that to parental rewards for good behavior.

10. Relate a preschooler's tendency to imitate adult behaviors to issues of safety.

Name: _____

Review

1. A 5-year-old child tries to pour juice from a heavy glass pitcher that he knows he is not supposed to touch. It slips from his hands and smashes on the floor and he bursts into tears. What negative feeling might Erikson say the child is experiencing?

    a. Shame
    b. Sadness
    c. Inferiority
    d. Guilt

2. What is the most likely explanation for accidental burns and poisonings in the preschool years?

    a. Aggressive behaviors
    b. Inability to understand reversibility
    c. Syncretic thinking
    d. Imitating parents

3. What stage of moral development is evident when a preschooler behaves only because they have been told that they will receive a reward?

    a. The golden rule
    b. Punishment and obedience
    c. Instrumental Purpose and Exchange
    d. Amorality

4. Which of the following best describes Piaget's intuitive stage of cognition?

    a. Having a gut feeling
    b. Use of memory and previous experience to aid in problem solving
    c. Having limited awareness of cause and effect
    d. Believing in absolutes

G&D: PRE-SCHOOL

PRE-SCHOOL Characteristics
- Physique – limbs & trunk proportional (small adult)
- Slower growth rate

Height increases only 2.5 – 3 inches/year;

Weight gain only 5 pounds/year

© MBWTE Photos, 2009

Images used under license from Shutterstock, Inc.

G&D: PRE-SCHOOL

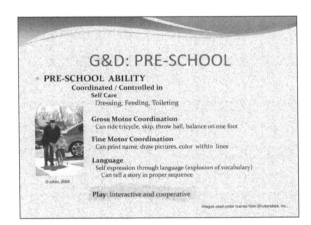

PRE-SCHOOL ABILITY
   Coordinated / Controlled in
       Self Care
           Dressing, Feeding, Toileting

   Gross Motor Coordination
       Can ride tricycle, skip, throw ball, balance on one foot

   Fine Motor Coordination
       Can print name, draw pictures, color within lines

   Language
       Self expression through language (explosion of vocabulary)
           Can tell a story in proper sequence

   Play: interactive and cooperative

© izfoto, 2009

Images used under license from Shutterstock, Inc.

G&D: PRE-SCHOOL

- **Pre-School Requirements:**
  - **Nutrition:**
    - Caloric needs minimal related to growth rate
    - Vitamins and minerals maximal related to energy level

  © Monkey Business Images, 200

  - **Oral Hygiene:** full set of 28 primary teeth
    - Need to brush and floss daily
    - Need to see Dentist x2/year

  - **Sleep:** 9-11 hours of sleep each night; may still take occasional nap in afternoon

Images used under license from Shutterstock, Inc.

G&D: PRE-SCHOOL

- **PRESCHOOL SAFETY**
  Car safety seats and seat belts
  Swimming safety equipment
  Helmets / Knee pads

  © Oxana Prokofyeva, 2009

  Supervision

  © Noam Armonn, 2009

  --love to impress adults (beware of **PREDATORS**)
    need to know to whom they can speak and when
    need to know that there should never be **secrets**
  - love to *imitate adults*
    (beware of knives, matches, medications,
    and alcohol)

  Images used under license from Shutterstock, Inc.

Know how to set Boundaries
→ Body Boundaries -
    -- correct touching by everyone

G&D: PRE-SCHOOL

- **PRE-SCHOOL PLAY**
  - Organized
  - Orchestrated (planned) yet Creative
    and Spontaneous
  - Interactive and Cooperative
    - With assigned roles and outcomes
    - Designated leaders and followers
  - Often imitative of adult roles
  - Often mixing reality with fantasy

  © MaszaS, 2009

  Images used under license from Shutterstock, Inc.

G&D: PRE-SCHOOL

PRE-SCHOOL PLAY
  Often involves *Art*
    resembling reality but don't ask
  Often involves *Music & Dance*
    more about rhythm than tone or style

  © Jacek Chabraszewski, 2009

  © Andi Berger, 2009

    May involve intermingling of reality
      with fantasy
    Having '*Imaginary Friends*' is
      perfectly normal

  Images used under license from Shutterstock, Inc.

G&D: PRE-SCHOOL

Pre-School Play vs. Pre-School Formalized Education

- *Play* (including board games) teach
  - Taking turns
  - Learning
  - Winning and Losing
  - Enjoyment of playing
    with less emphasis on competition

  © metka_Wananka, 2009

- *Formalized educational settings* often stifle
  - Creativity
  - Spontaneity
  - Individuality

Images used under license from Shutterstock, Inc.

G&D: PRE-SCHOOL

PRE-SCHOOL PSYCHOSOCIAL TASK – (Erikson)
INITIATIVE

- *Praise and encouragement*
  → feeling confident enough to perform actions independently,
    spontaneously, creatively
    → greater dependability, cooperation, assertiveness and
      organization
- *Ridicule and restrictions*
  → hesitancy to perform actions because it might not be right
  or feeling *guilty* for doing something wrong in the past.
    → assuming responsibility for actions that were not intended,
      This leads to even more hesitancy !

G&D: PRE-SCHOOL

PRE-SCHOOLERS NEED PRAISE

- Preschoolers thrive on *adult approval* –
  encouragement
  - Very different from bribery with money or candy or outings
  - Like to act like adults / help adults
  - Like to show off talents
  - Like to tell stories

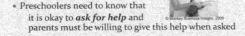

- Preschoolers need to know that
  it is okay to *ask for help* and   © Monkey Business Images, 2009
  parents must be willing to give this help when asked

Images used under license from Shutterstock, Inc.

G&D: PRE-SCHOOL

Pre-School Oedipal Complex
- This phenomenon occurs when
  - Pre-school children align themselves with the same sex parent and imitate them to such an extent that it sometimes becomes competitive especially when it is done to obtain the attention and affection of the opposite sex parent

- This phenomenon usually goes away by the time the child enters school

G&D: PRE-SCHOOL

PRE-SCHOOL COGNITION (Piaget)
- *INTUITIVE* (memory + beginning logical problem solving) – breaking cookie before attempting to 'dunk'   *logic*
- *CENTERED* – a boy is a boy; cannot be an uncle
- *ABSOLUTES* – girls have long hair;
                 boys have short hair
- *TRANSDUCTIVE* – general to general
  - a flower is a flower; cannot be a rose or tulip or carnation
  - a dog is a dog; not a chihuahua

G&D: PRE-SCHOOL

PRE-SCHOOL FEARS
- Some beginning Cause & Effect relating to consequences
  understand that some things may hurt them but
  don't understand how or why ⟶ FEAR
          boogey man
          dark
          animals
  Fears ⟶ Bedwetting, nightmares, sleepwalking

G&D: PRE-SCHOOL

- **LANGUAGE**
  - Vocabulary explosion (from 300 – 3000 words in a very short period of time)
  - Use complete sentences
  - Know correct tenses and can tell a story in proper sequence (and then...)
  - Know prepositions (on, under, behind, over)
  - Can describe objects
  - Can learn two or more languages simultaneously without confusion and/or mixing

G&D: PRE-SCHOOL

- **PRE-SCHOOL MORALITY** – (Kohlberg)
  - *Instrumental Purpose and Exchange*
    - What will I get / gain by doing this?
      - Parental approval and praise
      - A reward – money, toy, special treat
    - Learning how others feel
      - Understanding comfort, hurt, sharing

© Darren Whitt, 2009

Images used under license from Shutterstock, Inc.

G&D: PRE-SCHOOL

- **Pre-School Challenges**
  - *Sibling Rivalry*
    - Jealousy and resentment of perceived infringement of space, time, and affection from parents, usually from an older sibling towards a younger one, that may result in attempts to regain priority status
    - Requires parenting skill of dedicated time and attention
    - Need to acknowledge big girl/big boy differences in abilities

G&D: PRE-SCHOOL

- **Positive Parenting (Role Modeling) to minimize risk for**

Motor Vehicle Accidents / Pedestrian Accidents
- Safety seats and safety belts
- Crossing street safety guidelines

Respiratory illnesses
- Hand washing / Proper use of tissues
- Regular medical check-ups and Vaccines

Hearing and Vision Deficits
- Routine Screening

Injuries related to play and newly found independence
- Safe equipment, safe surfaces and protective equipment
- *SUPERVISION Essential*

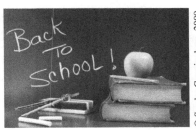

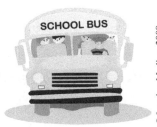

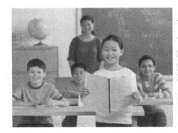

School Age (Age 6–12)

© Sandra Cunningham, 2009. Used under license from Shutterstock, Inc.

© Lorelyn Medina, 2009. Used under license from Shutterstock, Inc.

© AVAVA, 2009. Used under license from Shutterstock, Inc.

Objectives

Upon completion of this chapter, the reader should be able to:

1. Describe the physical characteristics of the school-age child.
2. Relate the physical abilities of the school-age child to safety recommendations.
3. Describe how Erikson's psychosocial task of Industry is best accomplished during the school-age years.
4. Describe how cognition (according to Piaget) relates to the elementary school curriculum.
5. Describe moral inclinations and capabilities (according to Kohlberg) that emerge during the school-age years.
6. Identify common illnesses and injuries that occur during the school-age years.
7. Describe parenting challenges as related to rearing the school-age child.

Key Terms

Classification: the cognitive ability to organize and group similar objects or information according to characteristics, such as size, color, or function

Concrete Operations: a level of cognition, according to Piaget, in which the thought processes are usually "hands on" and very "black and white." This is the level of cognition that is typical in school-age children.

Conservation of matter: a form of cognitive reversibility that recognizes that matter remains the same even though in different forms

Conventional Morality: morality based on the need to follow rules; "doing unto others what you would have them do unto you"

Industry: the psycho-social task for school-age children (according to Erikson) that is demonstrated by being successful at whatever is undertaken

Inferiority: a perception that one is not as good as others based on comparative feedback. Inferiority is the negative counterpart to Erikson's Industry.

Ordering: the cognitive ability to correctly organize information, such as numbers or letters, in a logical format

Ranking: the cognitive ability to prioritize objects by size or value or merit

Reversibility: the ability to recognize that some processes can be reversed, that is, undone

---

Physical and Physiological Characteristics

The school-age child (age 6–12) is usually slim and has longer legs than the preschooler. Most school-age children only gain around 6 pounds per year and increase their height by 2 inches per year. These are normal height and weight parameters but genetic predispositions definitely play a part. Generally speaking, boys and girls tend to be of similar height until the girls start their pre-pubescent growth spurt at around 10 to 12 years of age.

The school-age child has a mature GI system and can readily digest most foods. Because of the increased energy, there are increased caloric needs (up to 2400 calories/day) compared to the pre-school child. But dietary intake for the school-age child should be nutritious. Junk food has become so available and desirable that obesity in school-age children has become a definite problem of late. Currently over 9 % of school-age children are obese. Obesity is mostly related to overeating and/or eating unhealthy foods and to the absence or minimization of physical exercise.

The convenience and popularity of fast foods has contributed to obesity and limiting access to these foods is a definite parental challenge. Most schools have healthy eating programs to help parents and children make better choices and how to plan and prepare healthy meals. Schools also have physical education programs that are designed to develop and tone the muscles of school-age children in a fun setting.

Television and video games tend to preoccupy school-age children and minimize outdoor physical exercise. This, too, contributes to obesity. Obesity, as a precursor to high blood pressure and/or Diabetes, has become such a problem in school-age children that screenings are now routinely performed in many schools.

Elimination is usually not a problem for school-age children IF their diets are adequate and IF they take the time to let nature take its course. Constipation and/or enuresis sometimes occur when school-age children don't want to take time to completely empty their bowel and bladder. Unfortunately, this usually results in embarrassing accidents.

In the school-age child, there is increased neural myelinization that provides the school-age child with faster, quicker response times in their physical and mental abilities. They have great hand–eye coordination as evident in their ability to hit or kick a fast moving ball and in their ability to play the high-speed video games. School-age children also have quicker response time cognitively as evidenced by connectedness and integration of new learning.

Related to the increased muscle strength, school-age children are able to play longer and faster. Related to their increased cognitive ability to understand rules and roles, school-age children are quite capable of playing team sports. Team sports require cooperation, delayed gratification, and a healthy sense of competition. Most team sports for school-age children insist that ALL children have the opportunity to play, regardless of their ability, and stress sportsmanship rather than the win. Most schools and city leagues do not endorse teams that do not follow these standards.

There is increased density in the long bones and increased muscle mass, helping the school-age child acquire greater motor control, strength, flexibility, stamina, and endurance. But the bones are still growing and need to be protected. Protective helmets and arm and knee pads are critical to preserve the integrity of these growing bones as well as to prevent other more serious trauma.

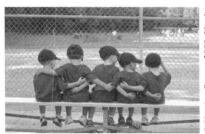 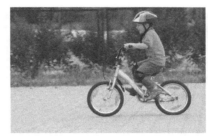 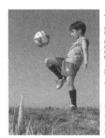

© Heather Renee, 2009. Used under license from Shutterstock, Inc.
© greenland, 2009. Used under license from Shutterstock, Inc.
© kristian sekulic, 2009. Used under license from Shutterstock, Inc.

Most school-age children have extremely large tonsils. Tonsils are a form of lymph gland that traps infection in the posterior pharynx before the infection settles into the lungs. There is also an increase in the size of other lymphoid tissues, indicating that the immune system is mature and active.

Most school-age children have lost their primary teeth and are seeing them replaced with larger secondary teeth. By 12 years of age, most children have a full set of 32 adult teeth. Since the secondary teeth will NOT be replaced, dental hygiene is critical during this time. Because secondary teeth are substantially larger, they often crowd one another and/or come in at awkward angles. It is not uncommon for school-age children to require orthodontics (braces) to straighten and better align their teeth.

The school-age child requires 10 to 12 hours of sleep. Sleep is necessary to allow the body to rest and recuperate, and also to allow the cells to grow. Too much activity and irregular sleep patterns sometimes result in nightmares, sleep talking, and/or sleep walking.

Safety Concerns

Because of their increased physical capabilities, school-age children often engage in activity that is beyond their ability. They often push themselves to excel in a skill to a point of injury especially when engaging in bicycle, skateboard, and all-terrain vehicle activities. School-age children also imitate adult behaviors and this could result in fire and firearm injuries, motor vehicle accidents, and drowning. As always, activities should be cautiously allowed and supervised when and where possible.

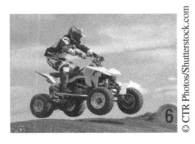 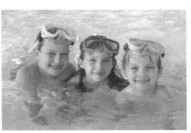 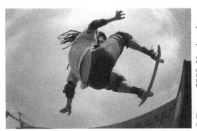

© CTR Photos/Shutterstock.com
© MaszaS, 2009. Used under license from Shutterstock, Inc.
© Ronen, 2009. Used under license from Shutterstock, Inc.

Developmental Theories

Industry vs. Inferiority (Erikson)

The psycho-social task for the school-age child, according to Erik Erikson (1968), is **Industry**. Industry, simply defined, is being capable and successful at whatever is undertaken and feeling significant and worthy because of this success. For school-age children, this applies to a multitude of activities. It is during the school-age period that children are expected to be successful in school (academic success), socialization (friendship success), individual and team sports (skill success), and music or dance (talent or aptitude success).

In the school setting, these children are expected to master reading, writing, basic mathematics, grammar, and spelling, as well as to become aware of global geography and historical events. School success (academics) is crucial to achieving *Industry*. School-age children love to brag about what they have learned and love to show parents and grandparents their accomplishments. This might be in grades on their report card or by having their "starred" paper placed on the refrigerator. For most school-age children, these undertakings are fun and they achieve a definite sense of pride when they accomplish them.

Healthy Competition

School-age children thrive on comparisons. If another school-age child can do it, they always want to do it even better. This is, for the most part, a healthy sense of competition. It is a personal challenge to be the BEST at everything they do. This sometimes takes the form of bragging not only about themselves, but about their relatives. For example, it is not uncommon to hear school-age children brag that "my dad is stronger than your dad" or "my mom can cook better than your mom."

Obviously, not everyone can be the best, and this sometimes creates an arena for frustration and a sense of **inferiority**. Parents and teachers need to recognize when their child is doing the best that THEY can, that this is all that should be expected. Children need to be praised for their effort and improvement in attempted tasks. To minimize the potential for frustration and/or feeling inferior, school-age children are generally praised and rewarded for the slightest success and/or improvement. At the end of school awards celebration, virtually everyone will receive an award for something, even if it is for having the "happiest smile."

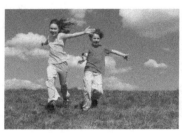
© Jacek Chabraszewski, 2009. Used under license from Shutterstock, Inc.

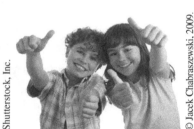
© Jacek Chabraszewski, 2009. Used under license from Shutterstock, Inc.

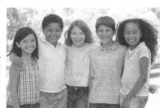
© Monkey Business Images, 2009. Used under license from Shutterstock, Inc.

Friendships

In friendship circles, school-age children strive to be liked by their peers. They want to be included in games and activities in and outside the classroom environment and want to feel that others want their company as well. School-age children, like most of us even in adulthood, try to impress others to achieve this inclusion. This might take the form of wearing stylish clothing, styling their hair a certain way, bragging about a gift they have received, or bragging about their parents. For others, it might take the form of being the "class clown" or being the smartest in the class or even by playing "dumb." For some school-age children, who truly do not have anything with which to impress others, they sometimes fabricate events and people just to get the attention that they so intensely desire. Lying is not uncommon during the school-age period. This will be discussed further under morality.

As in other tasks, school-age children are desperate to be the best in sports and music and dance. These should be fun activities that help the school-age child develop coordination, balance, strength, endurance, and socialization. These activities should not be about wins and losses, or recital and concert solos, or which person is the best in performing the skill. As in the classroom environment, these activities should encourage effort and achievement. In most team sports and in dance and music, children should be given full participation rights regardless of their natural abilities and should be equally rewarded.

For those students who struggle to master school-related subjects, and for those who are always the last to be picked to play on a team, and for those who are ignored on the playground or in social interactions, and for those who are uncoordinated in dance or who just can't get the hang of reading music, there is a strong sense of frustration and aloneness. The unsuccessful attempts of these children cause them to feel inferior. **Inferiority**, simply defined, is feeling less than adequate at expected tasks or feeling that one is not as good as others.

A challenge to parents is helping the child to realize their natural abilities and/or limitations. It is rare when a child is good at everything. Acknowledging effort is a good thing, but children need to learn that they usually are not the BEST at everything. A realistic perception of one's strengths and weaknesses is a challenge for all persons of all ages.

To minimize the risk for a school-age child to develop inferiority, parents are advised to guide their children to areas where success *can* be achieved. Sometimes school-age children are encouraged to participate in multiple activities like sports or music or dance. When the child is enjoying the wide range of activities, this is fine; but when they are struggling to sense any accomplishment, it might be better to allow them to concentrate on one activity in which they can either enjoy themselves or can be successful.

During the school-age period, children tend to desire friends of the same gender. Girls like to hang out with girls and to exclude boys. Boys, similarly, frequently post their "no girls allowed" signs. This is perfectly normal. Boy–girl attractions begin to occur when the pre-pubescent hormones kick in. This is usually around the age of 10 for girls and 14 for boys.

Concrete Operations (Piaget)

The cognition of the school-age child, according to Piaget (1950), is at a level of **Concrete Operations.** Concrete Operations is cognition in which the thought processes are usually driven by "hands-on manipulation," and involves simple, rule-oriented, direct, and black-and-white thinking. Abstract thought has not yet emerged. Things are what they are! This stage is characterized by tasks that involve **making things, ordering, classifying, ranking and reversibility.**

Hobbies

Hobbies are a characteristic trait of school-age children. They love to make simple things like model cars, buildings with erector sets, picture albums, pot holders, macramé lanyards, and key chains. This is all part of the increased ability to understand methodology and following instructions and they are rewarded for their efforts with a keepsake.

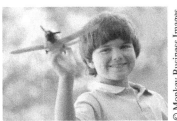

© Monkey Business Images, 2009. Used under license from Shutterstock, Inc.

© Tupungato/Shutterstock.com

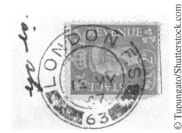

© Pavel Drozda, 2009. Used under license from Shutterstock, Inc.

Ordering is the ability to correctly organize information in a logical format, such as numbers or letters, and to perform tasks in proper sequence. Courses offered in the grade school curriculum are based on this ability because the school-age child understands the need to perform the step-by-step processes required in writing and basic math and can manipulate the numbers or words through reading and writing. School-age children are now able to put names or words in alphabetical order and spell words based on the phonetic pronunciations. They recognize that time is based on a 12 hour clock and know the difference between A.M. and P.M. School-age children can also understand that one nickel has more value than four pennies as compared to a pre-school child who would prefer *more* in terms of number of objects rather than value.

Classifying is organizing and nesting of information, that is, recognizing that similar objects can be grouped according to characteristics, such as size, color, make, or model. For example, understanding that sedans could be Chevrolets or Fords or other makes and that these are all cars. Another example would be to know that there are different types of leaves or blossoms on different types of trees. This is a definite progression from the pre-school limitation of centering. A typical hobby of school-age children is collecting items such as baseball cards, stamps, coins, and such, just so they can classify them.

Ranking is the ability to order in size or value or merit. For example, the school-age child can arrange numbers from large to small, arrange coins according to size or value, and recognize that earning an 'A' on a paper is better than getting a 'B'.

Reversibility is the ability to recognize that some processes can be reversed, i.e. undone. This is true in the basic math processes of addition and subtraction and in multiplication and division. **Conservation of matter** is a form of cognitive reversibility. School age children are able to understand that matter remains the same even though in different forms, e.g. water can be ice or steam but still be the same matter. Clay can be manipulated into different shapes, but it is still clay. Another classic example of conservation of matter is recognizing that volume does not change based on the size of the container. For example, if 4 ounces of water in a tall, thin glass is poured into a short fat glass, it is still 4 ounces of water. A pre-school child would think that the volume is less in the shorter glass.

School

The subjects taught in elementary school are purposefully designed to capitalize on the school age child's abilities to order, classify, rank and demonstrate reversibility. Learning to alphabetize and learning to spell are classic examples of ordering. Learning about historical events is also ordering. Learning where countries are located on a map is also an example of ordering and classifying. Reversibility is readily demonstrated in math when the child learns addition/subtraction and multiplication/division.

Impediments to Learning

It is often during the early school-age years that problems like attention deficit disorder and learning disabilities become apparent. In Attention Deficit Hyperactivity Disorder (ADHD), which for some reason, seems to be more prevalent in boys than in girls, there is an inappropriate degree of inattention, impulsiveness, and hyperactivity. Children with ADHD have difficulty paying attention to tasks in school, at home, and even during play. They do not seem to listen or follow through with instructions and rarely finish any project. In general, children with ADHD do not like activities that require sustained focus. They are easily distracted, do not pay attention to details, and are careless in their performance, that is, they appear very forgetful and often lose personal belongings. Many of these children act as if they are driven by a motor, that is, they are in constant motion or they talk excessively. ADHD children present a constant challenge to the patience of their parents and teachers and are often the ridicule of their classmates at school. Achieving "Industry" is extremely difficult for these children.

Impulsivity is also associated with ADHD. This causes children with this condition to blurt out answers before questions are complete and they often interrupt and/or intrude on other's conversations. Obviously these behaviors are NOT conducive to learning in an orderly classroom and furthermore the activities of

ADHD children inhibit the learning of children who do not have these tendencies. It is important to note that ADHD is NOT mental retardation. Many ADHD children have intelligence that is superior to others; they just cannot demonstrate it in a traditional classroom setting.

ADHD is generally treated with a combination of medication that helps the child to increase focus and with psychosocial communication therapy that helps the child to learn some behavior modifications. This combination therapy often allows the ADHD child to function in a regular classroom setting. But when the hyperactivity cannot be controlled, many of these children are educated in a more controlled environment in which there are fewer children and fewer distractions. These are "special education" classrooms.

Learning disabilities may also become apparent during the school-age years. With these disorders, children commonly interpret the order of numbers or letters in a reverse or scrambled manner that obviously causes them to have great difficulty in reading, spelling, mathematics, and with learning in general. These children definitely require individualized attention to help them figure out how to compensate for this erroneous interpretive tendency. It is similarly very difficult for these children achieve the psychosocial task of "Industry."

Conventional Morality (Kohlberg)

Morality, for the school age child, is described as **Conventional** by Kohlberg (1968). Conventional morality, simply defined, is 'doing unto others as you would have them do unto you'. Conventional morality is highly based on rules that everyone is expected to follow. A school age child becomes extremely frustrated when others do NOT follow rules in the classroom or at home or even in a game. School age children are notorious for tattle-telling on their peers because they did not follow the rules. As long as everyone follows the rules, there usually is no problem. Gilligan (1982) claims that it is during this stage that females exhibit more conditionality to behaviors. For example, Gilligan states that girls are more likely than boys, to understand that someone broke a rule for a good reason.

Did you know?

Did you know that school age children who are pressured to excel are more likely to engage in lying and cheating? The school age child who receives praise for doing the best they can has a realistic expectation of himself and is not inclined to inflate or camouflage his abilities.

Morality is of some concern during the school age years. Because the school age child is so desperate to feel successful, lying and cheating often occur. These children absolutely MUST be good at something, so they make it up or lie about their accomplishments. They may even resort to changing grades or copying school work because they want that good grade. Parents and teachers are challenged to correct these actions as soon as recognized.

Because most School age children are conformists to rules and to the expectations of society, deviance from these traits, known as conduct disorders, are usually very easy to detect. When children are overly aggressive or take on the role of 'bully', they obviously are not following the golden rule. Children with these tendencies take pleasure in threatening and/or inflicting pain on others and in destroying property. These are deliberate acts of cruelty and may include starting fires, destroying property, thievery, and lying. If identified and treated early on, these children can be rehabilitated with long-term psychotherapeutic counseling. But when there is no intervention or when treatment is delayed, the anti-social tendencies of these children tend to escalate into serious and life threatening physical acts of violence to both people and animals. Bullies, in general, tend to be suffering from inferiority. They need to control others in order to make themselves feel more important.

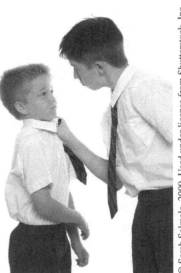

© Sarah Salmela, 2009. Used under license from Shutterstock, Inc.

Health Concerns

Physiologically, school age children are generally healthy. Nonetheless, they are vulnerable to upper respiratory infections and some other communicable conditions. Part of this is due to the fact that school age children are in such close contact with others and that they are exposed to an ever present array of multiple viruses and bacteria in the classroom environment. Most school age children also have not yet mastered the routine of frequent and thorough handwashing.

It is not uncommon for school age children to have extremely large tonsils. This does not mean that the tonsils need to be removed. It just means that the tonsils, as an integral part of the developing lymphatic system, are just doing what they were intended to do – trap infection before it descends into the lungs. With upper respiratory conditions, it is also common for school age children to have Otitis Media, a middle ear infection. The ear canal is still relatively short and straight and without the gravitational flow to the Eustachian tube and the lymphatic system, the infection tends to settle in the middle ear.

School age children are also vulnerable to contract communicable diseases such as measles, mumps, rubella and chicken pox. That is why it is so important that they receive the vaccines against these diseases before they enter school. Other common contagious conditions include Pink Eye and Pediculosis (head lice) and scabies. These are easily contracted in the school environment because children are less likely to be washing their hands as frequently as they should and are more likely to share combs, hats and scarves. These conditions are very treatable but tend to re-emerge because of the closely shared classroom environment.

Screening for hearing and vision is critical during the school age period because without optimal vision or hearing, students would not be able to be successful in their school work. Most schools schedule these screenings at least every other year.

Some psychological problems that become apparent during the school age period are depression and/or psychosomatic symptomatology (headache and stomach ache). Depression, characterized by withdrawing from others and sleep disturbances, is usually related to feelings of insecurity. These feelings may be a result of something going on at home like marital discord or physical or emotional abuse or it may be related to something going on at school like being bullied or not being accepted by their peers or teachers or coaches. School age children are intensely affected by these disruptive occurrences because they do not have the maturity to understand what is happening and they do not have the power or might to change these situations. This evokes fear and anxiety and becomes evident in behaviors like social isolation and/or having nightmares, sleep walking, and sleep talking.

The psychosomatic symptomatology of headaches and stomach aches may also be stress related but are generally linked more with the feelings of inferiority. These children become fearful of having that inferiority exposed when they are called upon to read out loud, or compete in a challenge or to take a test. Intervening on behalf of these children is necessary to help them identify what is bothering them and also to help them to cope with the issues in a more constructive manner.

Parental Concerns

Parents need to recognize that the school age child now has a whole new circle of acquaintances from whom they learn and share. In the pre-school years when the children were at home with only the parents, they did not know about what other children were allowed to do or to have or to say. Once they enter the school environment, it is all about comparing notes. Parents are encouraged to promote and encourage peer socialization but they also need to sustain home values, rules and priorities. Parents should always make family activities a priority over peer socialization.

Did you know that video games can actually help the school age child to increase eye-hand coordination? Video games can also help the school age child achieve a sense of accomplishment. Nonetheless, there is still a need to be selective in minimizing the extent of violence and there is still a need to limit the amount of time that is devoted to this activity.

Parental involvement in school or sports activities is highly encouraged. This helps parents to stay in touch with their own child in a new environment and allows parents to form their own parental support groups and opportunities for their socialization as well. Because of the unfortunate situation involving predators on young children, it is very challenging for parents to encourage outdoor exercise in the neighborhood because their home and work schedules preclude time for them to offer adequate supervision. This is why there are now so many team sports that allow the school age child to to get the exercise that they need.

Parents are also encouraged to limit the amount of time that their school age child spends watching TV or playing video games. While these activities can be educational and entertaining, school age children definitely need outdoor sunshine and physical exercise. They also need to have quiet time to read or to do their homework.

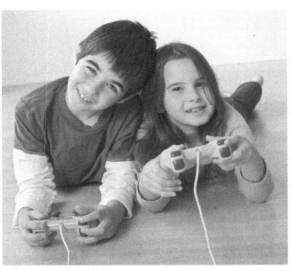

© Noam Armonn, 2009. Used under license from Shutterstock, Inc.

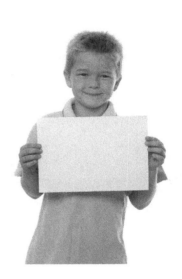

© Sarah Salmela, 2009. Used under license from Shutterstock, Inc.

The parenting skills required for the school age child are numerous. Parents should always remember to praise their child for any and all accomplishments and help the child to recognize and acknowledge their strengths. Industry can only be achieved when the child feels that they have been a success. All in all, most school age children are energetic in most activities, eager to learn and eager to please.

Summary

The school age child is full of energy, is eager to learn (loves school), is well coordinated, has endurance and stamina, is very social especially with members of the same sex, is highly competitive and absolutely must be good (successful) at something. They thrive on praise and encouragement and are generally speaking very happy individuals who just need support and direction in identifying their strengths.

References

Erikson, E. H. (1968) *Childhood and society* (35th anniversary edition). New York: Norton.

Gilligan, C (1982). *In a different voice: Psychological theory and women's development.* Cambridge, MA: Harvard University Press.

Kohlberg, L. (1969). *The philosophy of moral development: Vol. 1.* San Francisco: Harper & Row.

Piaget, J. (1950). *The psychology of intelligence.* London: Routledge and Kegan Paul.

Reflection

In the space below, recall what your success area was when you were a school age child. Describe how this success made you feel.

Assignment

Complete this form with essential data for School Age

Growth and Development Guide for School Age

	Physical Traits	Physical Abilities	Psychosocial Task (Erikson)	Evidence of How Achieved	Evidence of Non-Achievement	Cognitive Ability (Piaget)	Evidence of Achievement	Moral Capability (Kohlberg)	Evidence of Achievement
School Age (6–12 years)									

Study Guide for
School Age (6–12 Years)

1. Describe how and why the School Age child has better coordination, strength and stamina than the preschool child.

2. Explain why there are potential dangers associated with the school age child's increased physical ability.

3. Identify at least three ways in which a school age child might achieve Industry.

4. Identify at least three ways in which a school age child might experience Inferiority.

5. Explain what is meant by 'healthy' competition.

6. Explain why school is an ideal setting for achieving Industry and for accomplishing Concrete Operations.

7. Compare and contrast the understanding of 'centering', 'cause and effect' and 'time' between a school age child and a pre-schooler.

8. Describe what is meant by the following terms and give an example of each:

   Classifying

   Ranking

   Reversibility

   Conservation of Matter

9. How do hobbies and crafts help a school age child accomplish Concrete Operations?

10. Describe what is meant by the 'Golden Rule' and explain why rules are so important to a school age child.

Name: _____`

Review

1. Which of the following is most characteristic of conventional morality?

    a. insisting that everyone follow the rule
    b. talking when the teacher is not looking; stopping when teacher turns around
    c. bringing a present to the teacher in order to get a better grade
    d. thinking about why someone may have been 'bad' rather than focusing on the action

2. Which of the following BEST describes socialization during the school age years?

    a. Same sex friendships are preferred.
    b. Boys and girls do not indicate gender preferences in selecting friends.
    c. Boys generally start showing interest in girls around age 8.
    d. Girls generally start showing interest in boys around age 7.

3. Which of the following is most likely a contributing reason for lying and/or cheating during the school age years?

    a. Need to be the best at something
    b. Ineffective parenting
    c. Golden rule morality
    d. Social exclusion

4. Which of the following conditions is most likely the result of sharing clothes or combs?

    a. Scabies
    b. Pediculosis
    c. Influenza
    d. Otitis media

G&D: SCHOOL AGE

SCHOOL AGE Physical Characteristics
- Slim with longer legs than the preschooler
- Weight gain: Six (6) pounds per year
- Height increase: Two (2) inches per year.

  (Boys and girls tend to be of
  similar height until the girls
  start their pre-pubescent
  growth spurt at around
  10 – 12 years of age.)

© Monkey Business Images, 2009

Images used under license from Shutterstock, Inc.

G&D: SCHOOL AGE

SCHOOL AGE Physical Characteristics
- Large tonsils (growth of lymphatic system)
- Losing primary teeth and gaining secondary teeth
  - Dental care related to
    - Caries
    - Braces – larger secondary teeth
- Mature GI system
  - can readily digest most foods
  - usually do not have problems with elimination

© Monkey Business Images, 2009

Images used under license from Shutterstock, Inc.

G&D: SCHOOL AGE

SCHOOL AGE Requirements
- **Nutrition**
  - Increased caloric needs (up to 2400 calories /day)
    - related to energy level but
    - dietary intake should be nutritious rather than 'junk' food
  - Currently over 11% of school age children are *obese*
    - overeating and/or eating unhealthy foods and
- **Exercise**
    - absence or minimization of physical exercise
      - Video games contributing?
- **Sleep** – 10-12 hours of sleep each night

G& D: SCHOOL AGE

SCHOOL AGE Physical Characteristics

Increased myelinization of neural pathways ⟶

Faster response in physical and mental abilities

Improved *muscle tone* and coordination

Improved *eye-hand coordination*

Increased *Strength* and *Endurance*

© Larry Maurer, 2018

© Noam Armonn, 2009

Images used under license from Shutterstock, Inc.

G&D: SCHOOL AGE

SCHOOL AGE Physical Characteristics

- Increased density in long bones and increased muscle mass ⟶ motor control, strength, flexibility, stamina
- But bones are still growing and need to be protected. Protective helmets and arm and knee pads are critical to preserve the integrity of these growing bones as well as to prevent other more serious trauma.

© greenland, 2009

Images used under license from Shutterstock, Inc.

G&D: SCHOOL AGE

SCHOOL AGE Physical Characteristics

- **Safety:** protective equipment; realistic expectations
- **Supervision**
  - Often think they can do more than they realistically can

© Marcel Jancovic, 2011

© Andi Berger, 2009

© Ronah, 2009

Images used under license from Shutterstock, Inc.

G& D: SCHOOL AGE

Psychosocial Task (Erikson) of *Industry*
- Need to achieve; need to be good at something
  - School, Friends, Sports, Skills, Music, Art, Dance

Opposing sense of *Inferiority* occurs when
- Not liked, not successful

Parental Challenge to help children to find strengths
without making them feel Inferior or overwhelmed

Images used under license from Shutterstock, Inc.

G&D: SCHOOL AGE

- **SCHOOL**
  - Perfect environment for gaining INDUSTRY
  - Is task oriented
  - Is hands on (black and white)
  - Involves memory
  - Generates rewards
    - Stars
    - Refrigerator posters
    - Bragging rights
    - Sense of pride: "MOST IMPROVED"...

© AVAVA, 2009

Images used under license from Shutterstock, Inc.

G& D: SCHOOL AGE

- Industry
  - COMPARISON (must be BEST)
  - COMPETITION but
  - being a TEAM MEMBER is necessary
    - for social development

© Heather Renee, 2009

Socialization helps school age children
learn give and take. Unfortunately, some
school age children who feel inferior,
resort to bullying to sustain self-esteem

© Veronica Louro, 2016

Images used under license from Shutterstock, Inc.

G&D: SCHOOL AGE

- School Age Children prefer friends of the same sex but are friendly with both genders
  - Hormonal influences do not enter the picture until around age 10 for girls; 14 for boys

© Monkey Business Images, 2009

© Jacek Chabraszewski, 2009

Images used under license from Shutterstock, Inc.

G&D: SCHOOL AGE

- School Age Children thrive on being 'liked' and accepted by peers
  - Included in games / parties
  - Tend to dress alike / talk alike
  - Compare parental rules and expectations

© Jacek Chabraszewski, 2009

- INFERIORITY
  - Unliked
  - Last picked for games
  - Unsuccessful in School, Sports, Music, etc.

Images used under license from Shutterstock, Inc.

G& D: SCHOOL AGE

- Cognition (Piaget) *Concrete Operations*
  - Hobbies – a major component of concrete operations
  - Collections like stamp collections / baseball cards

© Monkey Business Images, 2009

© Marek Slusarczyk, 2009

- Crafts / building/creating

Images used under license from Shutterstock, Inc.

about here & now / Not so much future.

G&D: SCHOOL AGE

- Cognition (Piaget) *Concrete Operations*
  - Hands on / black and white learning – this is what makes school so much fun and interesting
    - Ordering: ability to organize in logical sequence
    - Memory: learning states / capitals / historical facts
    - Classification: organizing and nesting of information into categories / understanding parts of speech / grammar
    - Sorting: stamps / collections of baseball cards
    - Ranking by quantity and quality
    - Reversibility – Conservation of matter
      - multiplication tables / learning division

G&D: SCHOOL AGE

- Other children suffer with learning and/or behavioral deficits
  - Attention Deficit Hyperactivity Disorder (ADHD)
    - lack focus –treatable but difficult for a child to develop the essential task of Industry
  - Learning disabilities
    - distort spatial placement of words on a page or
    - make number calculations extremely difficult –
    - remedied with specialized educational interventions
  - Gaining a sense of INDUSTRY extremely difficult for children with these deficits

G&D: SCHOOL AGE

- School Age Morality (Kohlberg) is **Conventional**
  - Golden Rule
    - Beginning of understanding how events impact others
    - Most School Age children are GOOD
      - Bullies and Deviants easy to detect
  - Also driven to be BEST
    - Results in lying & cheating for success and/or bragging rights
    - Lying because of not wanting to be considered 'bad'
    - Bullying
    - Understanding that order is necessary for the larger good
  - Insist that Rules must be obeyed –
    - Sometimes results in tattle tale syndrome

G&D: SCHOOL AGE

* Common School Age Medical Concerns

Head lice → Pediculosis / Mites
* Respiratory contagious conditions: colds, flu, otitis media – vaccines essential
* Pinkeye
* Alterations in hearing and vision – screening essential
* Psychosomatic symptoms of headache and stomach ache usually related to
  * Problems at home
  * Problems in the classroom

G& D: SCHOOL AGE

* Parenting of School Age Child
  * Involvement in School and extracurricular activities
  * Praise and encouragement helps them to succeed
  * Realistic Expectations – help them to find strengths; recognize weaknesses
  * Supervise and Protect
    * Safety concerns related to increased abilities and eagerness to excel
    * Injury concerns related to protecting growing bones

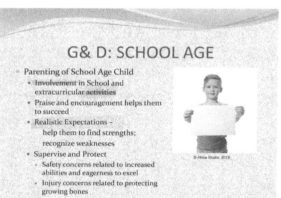

© Africa Studio, 2018

Images used under license from Shutterstock, Inc.

Adolescence (Age 12–18)

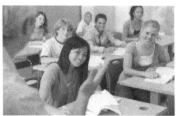

© Monkey Business Images, 2009. Used under license from Shutterstock, Inc.

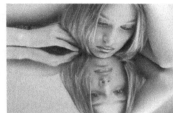

© Bliznetsov, 2009. Used under license from Shutterstock, Inc.

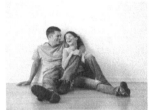

© iofoto, 2009. Used under license from Shutterstock, Inc.

Objectives

Upon completion of this chapter, the reader should be able to:

1. Describe the dramatic growth changes that occur during adolescence.
2. Describe the nutritional and sleep demands on the body related to the growth changes during adolescence.
3. Compare and contrast the physiologic and psychological characteristics of the adolescent with those of younger aged individuals.
4. Define and differentiate *adolescence* and *puberty*.
5. Explain the role of peers in the development stage of adolescence.
6. Define *identity* as described by Erikson and describe the tasks associated with achieving identity.
7. Define *formal operations* as described by Piaget and describe the limitations of this cognitive ability during adolescence.
8. Describe the parental challenges associated with rearing an adolescent.
9. Identify common concerns, illnesses, and injuries associated with adolescence.

Key Terms

Adolescence: the stage of development associated with psychological and emotional maturation into adulthood

Body dysmorphia: a distorted perception of body image that causes individuals to engage in unhealthy drastic action in order to achieve a body image more in keeping with their ideal

Fable of immunity: an unrealistic perception by many teens that causes them to believe that even though bad things can and do happen to others, these things won't happen to them

Formal Operations: Piaget's stage of cognition that is characterized by the ability to formulate hypotheses and possible solutions, that is, the ability to think about thinking and to think abstractly.

Gender Identity: recognizing and accepting the gender with which an individual is comfortable in practicing everyday activities whether or not it is the gender to which they were born.

Identity: the stage of development, as described by Erikson, during which individuals recognize their uniqueness in role and accountability and act accordingly

LGBT orientation: Lesbian, Gay, Bi-sexual, Transgender sexual orientation

Menarche: first menses

Peer pressure: the effect of influence of friends on choices related to dress, speech, and behavior

Puberty: the stage of development associated with the physiologic changes that occur during adolescence. Puberty begins with the appearance of secondary sex characteristics and ends with the closure of the epiphysis of the long bones and the maximizing of height.

Role confusion: the inability of an individual to differentiate themselves as unique resulting in a period of discontent and nondescript behaviors

Scoliosis: a curvature of the spinal column that may result from rapid growth. Scoliosis is often associated with mobility aberrations, joint pain, and displaced internal organs.

Secondary sex characteristics: non-reproductive body changes associated with hormonal influences that occur during adolescence. Examples include deepening of the voice and growth of facial hair in the male, breast development and spreading of the pelvis in females.

Wet dream: a spontaneous emission of ejaculate during sleep that may or may not be associated with an erotic dream; a sign of male sexual maturation, that is, puberty

---

Adolescent Physical Growth Spurt (Puberty)

Other than during infancy, there is no other age frame in which growth is so rapid and diverse than in adolescence. Females experience the growth spurt associated with adolescence earlier than males. Girls increase in height 4 to 6 inches during this surge of growth and it is not uncommon at all to see girls towering over the boys in 5th or 6th grade (approximately 10–12 years of age). This is called a prepubescent growth spurt because it is associated with the pubescent changes that are about to occur.

Unfortunately, with the prepubescent growth spurt, especially in females, is the increased risk for scoliosis. **Scoliosis** is curvature of the spine that may be of genetic origin or a result of rapid asynchronous growth. Scoliosis may cause the preteen to experience increased hip or knee pain, to lean to one side or to walk with a limp, but the greatest concern with scoliosis is associated with the displacement of internal organs that in turn cause increased pressure on the heart and lungs. Scoliosis, when detected early, can be repaired with bracing and surgical intervention. But it is important to make these corrections BEFORE growth is complete, because, once the bones stop growing, they are much more difficult to realign.

Following this increase in height is the appearance of **secondary sex characteristics**. These characteristics are called secondary because they are not primarily associated with sexual reproduction. For females, the

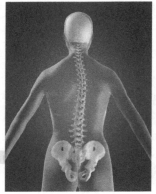

© Sebastian Kaulitzki, 2009. Used under license from Shutterstock, Inc.

first evidence of secondary sex characteristics is usually the breast bud followed by full breast development. Another secondary sex characteristics for the female is the widening of the pelvis.

These two physiologic changes are purposeful as well as giving females a more shapely appearance. The breasts have developed to prepare the body for breast feeding of an infant and the hips have widened to facilitate the expansion of the pelvis during pregnancy and the delivery of a baby through the birth canal. Other secondary characteristics of the female include growth of pubic and underarm hair.

Following the appearance of these prepubescent characteristics is usually the onset of menses. **Menarche**, the first menses, is indication that the female body has reached **puberty**, that is, the maturation of sexual reproductive ability. Once menses has occurred, females are physiologically capable of conceiving and bearing a child. It is another story about whether or not they are psychologically or emotionally mature enough to handle this situation.

It has been found that the onset of menses (menarche) is linked with body fat proportion. Females with greater fat proportion tend to start their menstrual cycle earlier than females who are leaner. It is interesting to note that females with very lean proportions, (gymnasts, for example) usually do NOT experience the growth prepubescent changes or menarche until 14 or 15 years of age.

The onset of menses is also usually the end of the growth spurt for females. The epiphyses of the long bones close and so maximum height is achieved. No further increases in height will occur after this time.

Males, typically, do not experience their growth spurt until around age 14 or 16. One of the first indications is that of a noticeable increase in shoe size. The feet grow first to sustain the increased length that is about to occur in the long bones of the legs. It is not uncommon to see an increase in clumsiness during this stage such as stumbling over their own feet. For most males, there is also a noticeable increase in the size and tone of the muscles in their arms and legs.

The secondary sex characteristics that then become apparent in males include deepening of the voice; growth of facial, pubic, and underarm hair; and enlargement and elongation of the penis and testes.

Puberty is complete for the male when the reproductive organs, the testes, reach full maturation. This maturation is evident with the emission of the first ejaculate. The first ejaculate usually occurs during sleep and is often referred to as a **wet dream**. When wet dreams occur, it is incorrect to assume that this occurred as a result of an erotic fantasy or dream. This can and does occur spontaneously.

As with females, the evidence of sexual reproductive maturation in males is also evidence that they have the capability of fathering a child. Once again, this does not mean that they are psychologically or emotionally mature to deal with becoming a parent.

Did you know?

Did you know that the average age of menarche has become younger over the last 50 years? Do you think that young females weigh more now than they did 50 years ago?

Hormones

The physiological changes associated with puberty are the result of hormonal influences. Hormones, body secretions of the endocrine system, are responsible for the activation of the secondary sex characteristics, and for the maturation of the sexual organs of reproduction. For females, the primary hormone is estrogen and for males, the primary hormone is testosterone.

The raging hormones are responsible for strong physical and sexual attraction to other individuals.

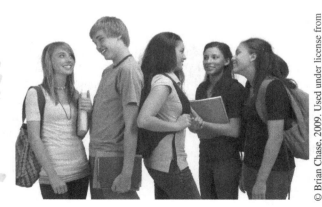

The girls and boys that have been shunned during earlier school years are now found to be cute and most desirable. At first there is a lot of teasing and flirting and just hanging out. Then, when the attraction becomes especially singular, dating begins. Dating is a healthy way for teenagers to understand their own sexuality and to establish meaningful relationships with others. When teens value and respect themselves and value and respect the individuals whom they are dating, it is a very good scenario. It is during this time that teens can explore what they like or dislike about members of the opposite sex or members of the same sex in preparation for finding a life partner.

In dating, teens learn about interpersonal communication and how to mutually agree to disagree. They also learn a lot about give-and-take negotiations. Teens, unfortunately, very often engage in sexual exploration before relationships are firmly established.

Sexual experimentation is very common during adolescence. Whether it is heterosexual or bi-sexual or homosexual or transgender, sexuality is a major issue during adolescence. It is a very difficult time for teens because they are experiencing so many hormonal changes and they do not know how to respond. It is even more difficult for teens who recognize that their hormonal attractions do not necessarily coincide with their birth gender. These teens, with gender identity concerns, find themselves in a very lonely world. They don't fit the mold and/or the expectations that go with it. Whether they are of lesbian, homosexual, bisexual, or transgender orientation, it is extremely difficult for them to establish their own identity.

When it comes to hormones vs. reason, the hormones will usually win. The best one can hope for is that teens will not engage in sexual activity until they are ready and will be discriminating about when and with whom this occurs. Discussions about responsible sexual activity that address self-esteem, respect, protection, and prevention should be ongoing.

Teens commonly confuse sex with love and affection. Individuals with high self-esteem learn that love and affection can be achieved through friendships and loyalties that do not necessarily involve sex. But individuals who are struggling for identity (high self-esteem) perceive sex differently. Even though sex may only provide momentary pleasure, it usually also provides a momentary attention that is craved and as Maslow (1968) indicates, we all want and need love and affection.

It is not so much the act of sex that is the concern; it is the consequences of sex that are so devastating. Experimenting with sexual activity is a major concern during the teen years. Teens are not only capable of having sex but are quite capable of conceiving and bearing children and communicating serious sexually transmitted diseases. What teens are not capable of is the full understanding of these implications and potential consequences.

Did you know?

Did you know that in most states, teens can receive health care related to sexually transmitted disease and contraception without parental permission? The problem is that the teens may not have access to these clinics and even if they do, they cannot afford to pay for services on their own.

Unfortunately, despite numerous strategies to address healthy perspectives of sex among teenagers, pregnancy and sexually transmitted disease have a sustained prevalence among teens. Chlamydia, the number one sexually transmitted disease among all sexually active individuals, has an alarming high rate among teens. And oral chlamydia is becoming even more prevalent in this age group. Teen pregnancy, though sustainable, is always considered high risk because of the teen's tendency to experiment with other risky behaviors (like substance abuse) and to have poor nutrition. Teen parents are forced to forego the freedoms experienced by their peers and are forced into a role designed for a more mature, responsible adult. The children born to teens are also at high risk for low birth weight, prematurity, and child abuse.

Other hormones become active during the teen years as well. Secretions from the eccrine and appocrine sebaceous glands result in increased perspiration and are also responsible for the clogging of skin pores that may result in acne. Both scenarios require greater attention to hygiene. More frequent bathing and the use of deodorants are a must for most teenagers.

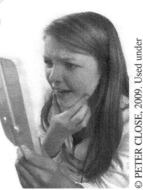

Despite the many myths about colas and chocolate causing and/or exacerbating acne, there is no researched evidence that this is true. Acne is hormonal in origin. Some individuals may have a greater susceptibility to acne related to genetic predisposition, but dietary choices have not been shown to influence the outcome. Some over-the-counter remedies may help control acne but some products merely cover it up, and tend to make it worse by clogging the pores even more. Popping pimples to squeeze out the exudate is not recommended. This practice, more often than not, results in infection. Hygiene, proper cleansing with soap and water, is still the best preventive practice and remedy. If acne is excessive and/or becomes infected, it is recommended that the teen seek the help of a dermatologist.

Health Maintenance

Because of the tremendous changes in physiologic growth, the adolescent body demands optimal nutrition and optimal sleep. Unfortunately, both requirements are often ignored by teenagers. Teenagers require up to 10 hours of sleep each night but most get less than 7 hours. Some of this is related to the increased hours of study demanded for academic success and some is related to increased activities outside of school. This may be sports, work, or simply a desire to just hang out with their friends. Nonetheless, the growing body of a teenager needs sleep. It is not uncommon for many teenagers to catch up on their sleep by sleeping in late on the weekends.

Nutrition is often deficient in the lives of most teenagers. Because of their increased involvement in school, work, sports, and other activities, teens rarely eat balanced meals. Adolescents are also sufficiently independent to choose the foods that they prepare and eat. Unfortunately, most choose to eat fast food that is very low in nutrient value and high in fat and empty calories.

Body Image

The physiological body changes that occur during the teen years are often a source of psychological disturbance. A positive body image is crucial to feeling good about oneself and attractive to others. For this reason, an excessive amount of attention is given to the way the teen looks. Teens are extremely aware of and critical of the changes in their bodies. If they are happy with the changes, there is usually no problem. But if their body is not maturing at the same rate as their peers or if the end result is less desirable than what they want, many teens become overly preoccupied with the comparisons and often exhibit psychologically negative responses. It is essential that teens perceive themselves with a healthy and realistic body image.

This is why teens spend an enormous amount of time in front of the mirror, preening and readjusting to meet the eye of their beholders. This is why teen styles, often described by adults as eccentric, are so eagerly adopted. Whether a particular clothing style is classic or weird to adults, it is what is accepted in the social circle of friends in which they want to be and that is what matters most. Peer acceptance is also apparent in the way teens wear their hair, walk, and talk. It is like there is an established protocol that must be followed. This code of conduct can be positive or negative. This becomes even more apparent when dating begins.

While most teens probably perceive their bodies as less than perfect at one time or another, most are eventually able to accept what nature has given them. Other teens cannot accept the changes or lack thereof in their bodies.

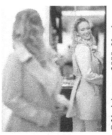

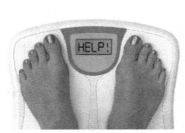

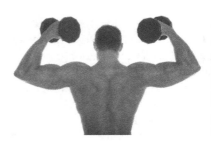

This results in a perceived body dysmorphia. **Body dysmorphia** is simply a distorted perception of body image. When individuals perceive themselves as weighing more than their peers or when they perceive themselves as wimpy in musculature, they often engage in unhealthy drastic actions in order to achieve their perceived "ideal" body image. These actions may include eating disorders, excessive physical exercise, and/or use of steroids.

Eating disorders, more commonly found in females than in males, include anorexia nervosa and bulimia. Anorexia nervosa is a condition in which individuals refuse to eat or eat minimally because they want to lose weight or want to keep from gaining any weight. This obviously results in severe nutritional deficits, anemia, muscle wasting, dehydration, and hypertension. When continued over an extensive period of time, this could result in cardiac and/or renal failure.

Bulimia is a condition in which individuals purge themselves of consumed food so that it doesn't cause them to gain weight. Purging is usually accomplished by inducing vomiting and in some cases includes the excessive use of laxatives, enemas, and/or diuretics. Bulimia also results in similar nutritional deficits as described above for anorexia nervosa.

Purging, for many individuals, becomes habitual no matter how much or how little food has been eaten. In other cases, purging follows a food binge. A food binge occurs when an individual consumes an excessive amount of food. This often occurs after extreme fasting. Following the binge, the individual feels so guilty about eating so much that they feel compelled to get rid of the potential weight gain. Purging, besides being nutritionally unsound, often causes severe physiological trauma. Related to the acidic content in the reflux there can be extensive damage to the lining of the esophagus and oral cavity and serious erosion of the tooth enamel.

The exercise-based body dysmorphias are more commonly seen in males who perceive themselves as wimpy compared to their peers. These individuals will spend hours and hours weight lifting and toning muscles and/or using steroids to improve their own body image. Intense and heavy weight lifting before puberty has been found to cause excessive stress on the long bones and joints and may eventually stunt growth. The use of steroids, besides being illegal, has commonly been associated with cardiac and renal problems and has also been associated with male impotence.

Body dysmorphias obviously impact negatively on physiological well–being, but it is the psychological damage that has the more serious long-term effects. Most individuals engaging in body dysmorphia activities require prolonged psychotherapy to overcome their distorted body image.

Emotional Maturation (Adolescence)

In conjunction with dealing with the multiple and rapidly changing physiological changes, teens are also challenged to mature psychologically and emotionally. **Adolescence** is the very vague term associated with the teen years that addresses the psychological and emotional maturation into adulthood. Adolescence is not as automatic as the physiological hormonal changes and cannot be as predictable in sequence as is puberty. Adolescence also cannot be limited to a specified age.

The psychological changes commonly associated with adolescence are also driven by hormones. These hormones, because they are not yet regulated by a mature feedback mechanism, are often extremely labile.

This is why teens are sometimes described as acting like an old man or woman and at other times described as acting like a 2-year-old. Teens tend to be very emotional. They laugh and cry easily. They can be on top of the world one minute and very depressed in the next minute. Teens tend to be quickly swayed for or against policies and are avid in pursuing and promoting these causes. These mood swings are extremely challenging to parents and teachers and are quite disturbing to the teens themselves.

Developmental Theories

Identity vs. Role Confusion (Erik Erikson)

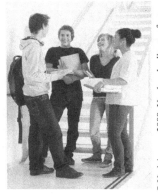

© Yuri Arcurs, 2009. Used under license from Shutterstock, Inc.

During adolescence, teens are expected to figure out who they are, who they will be, what they will be doing in the future, and where they will be going. If successful in achieving this task, according to Erikson (1968), individuals possess identity. **Identity**, simply defined, is recognizing one's uniqueness in role and accountability and then acting accordingly. This is a huge task and does not spontaneously occur. Identity hopefully will evolve over the course of the teen years but is rarely seen in young teens. Some individuals fail to accomplish this task during their teen years. When this occurs, the teens are said to be in **role confusion**, a period of non-descriptive, non-direction, and discontent with themselves and life in general.

Peer acceptance is crucial to the formation of identity. This almost seems paradoxical to say that we need others to know who we are but it is true. It is through others that we know ourselves. It is because of the positive or negative reactions of others that we develop certain behaviors. We learn early in life how to put on our clothes right side out and to tie our shoes. But it is through the reactions of others that we learn what really looks "good" on us, what really goes together well and what is in or out of style.

Peer acceptance is especially difficult for those with gender identity issues. Even though LGBT support is now more apparent in society in general, this may or may not be apparent within a teen's circle of friends or even within their own family.

To achieve identity, teens need a strong basis of support and guidance. Parents, who have been their strongest support up to this point in their life, suddenly are not perceived nearly as credible and certainly not as important as their peers. It is their friends to whom they cling for insight and perspective.

Peer pressure is the term often used to describe the extent of influence by persons of the same age, gender, and experience that is evident in personal choices and behavior. A major parenting challenge is to guide teens to a good choice of friends. If a teen's friends are good, they generally will be too. If the teen's friends are into "not so good" activities, it is very likely that the teen will follow their example.

Peer pressure can be very positive. Because friends are volunteering time to build homes and serve meals for the homeless, a teen may opt to participate in these activities as well. The fact that friends are getting good grades in school may inspire a teen to stay competitive with them and be successful as well. But often peer pressure is negative and influences teens to participate in activities that are less than desirable. Many teens engage initially in these negative activities only to impress their friends or to prove that they are like them and desperately want to be accepted by them.

Teens experiencing **role confusion** tend to follow the convenient crowd. These crowds are usually not engaged in positive purposeful activity and are often involved in truancy, bullying, substance abuse, indiscriminate sexual activity, violence, and vandalism. Gangs that are formed during adolescence are typical of this type of behavior.

Another concern, sometimes linked with peer pressure is the urge for many teens to engage in the exploration of what they perceive as adult privilege. This may be in drinking alcohol or smoking or taking drugs.

Fortunately, many do not like the effects and choose not to persist in these behaviors. Others establish a pattern of behavior that becomes habituated and very difficult to stop. As with most bad habits, it is always best NOT to get started in the first place but this is a very difficult concept for teens.

Peer acceptance is important in all stages of life but it carries less significance once identity has been achieved. **Identity** is evident when individuals have sufficient confidence in themselves to act independently of the group. Individuals possessing identity have a strong sense of self-esteem. They do not fear rejection by their friends and are less dependent on the approval of others. So, when teens feel confident that their friends will still be friends even though they don't go with them to a ball game or when they choose to participate in an activity not particularly favored by their friends, they have found their own uniqueness and are not afraid to show it. Teens with high self-esteem and identity are more likely to be successful in life and less likely to engage in risky behaviors.

Cognition: Formal Operations (Piaget)

Even though teens have the cognitive ability to think abstractly, they often think they know more than they actually do. This coupled with lack of experience often results in errors of judgment. So no matter what adults may tell them about potential dangers, teens tend to have a false sense of immunity from bad effects. This is known as the **fable of immunity**. This means that they are aware that alcohol and pot smoking has caused diminished brain function in others, but they have things "under control" so these bad effects will not happen to them. This same sort of misconception may cause them to drive while intoxicated, speed while driving, and have sex without protection.

Many of the concerns related to adolescence center around the teen's perception. This is related to their cognitive ability. According to Piaget (1950), teens at about the age of 13 are capable of formal operations. **Formal operations** is the highest order of thinking in Piaget's schema and indicates that individuals can think abstractly, can think about thinking, and can hypothesize about problems and potential solutions. But teens do not have the life experiences to make formal operations fully operational.

Education is only one aspect of formal operations. Even after completion of a college degree, there are limitations in the extent of formal operations cognition. It is often quoted that as many as 30% of adults never reach the stage of full formal operations cognition.

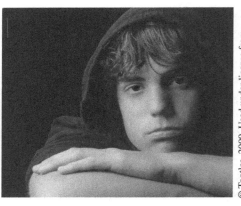

© Tootles, 2009. Used under license from Shutterstock, Inc.

Teens tend to very introspective and analyze and criticize themselves deeply. For example, rejection by peers or a member of the opposite sex or experiencing a breakup in a dating relationship can make a teen feel totally undesirable and unloved. Gender identity issues have greatly added to this self-loathing.

Depression among adolescents is a form of role confusion in the struggle to find identity. This is not uncommon, but in some extreme cases, this depression has resulted in suicide and this is becoming more and more apparent. Parents and teachers need to be alert to prolonged periods of aloneness and/or symptoms of apathy. If these signs are apparent, parents and teachers need to directly confront the teen about their thoughts and refer them for professional intervention immediately. Erring on the side of caution is always preferred. Deferring referral when symptoms are present should never be an option.

Limited exposure to the realities of life often causes the adolescent to be very idealistic and overly critical of others. They may be able to understand some aspects of the two sides of an issue but tend to adhere strongly to one or the other. They are not exactly easily swayed but once they are convinced, it is very difficult for them to consider an alternative.

Morality: Social System and Development of Conscience (Kohlberg)

Because of the increased ability in cognition to analyze situations, adolescents are now more aware of their surroundings and the need for establishing some order in the midst of chaos. This is part of the reason that they take on causes so readily and avidly.

Nonetheless, adolescents also tend to reject the status quo. Just because things have always been done a certain way is the very reason why teens think they should NOT be done this way. It is not uncommon for adolescents to reject politics, religion, and family values. This is why parents often lose credibility. If parents have not been successful in convincing their teen of a value or ideal at an earlier age, it certainly will not work now. Parents can no longer use rationale like "because I said so." Unless there is sound evidence when stating facts, teens will scoff and ignore them.

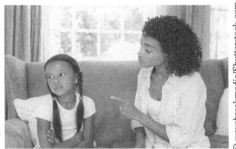

© wavebreakmedia/Shutterstock.com

Parental Challenges

This is not to say that parents cannot or should not enforce rules. Teens need structure and this is commonly experienced through rules. But parents also need to know that rules are going to be broken and parents must be able to live with that fact as well. Parents should also be encouraged to choose their battles. Not all issues need to take on mega proportions. It is in the nature of a teenager who is striving to attain identity and independence that they will test the limits of rules. That is why consequences must fit the offense, and must be clearly stated when the rules are put into force. That way if a teen chooses to break the rules, they must also learn to accept the consequences. And parents absolutely need to enforce the consequences. When parents do not enforce the consequences, the rules and the parents will no longer be respected.

The adolescent needs to experience some independent judgment and parents should encourage them to make independent choices. Hopefully values that have been instilled at an earlier stage will guide these choices. Rules should only be for undesirable activities and should absolutely be limited. Too many rules become control and this just creates a hostile environment that will surely elicit revolt.

Rules also serve as safety nets and boundaries. Even though many teens have told their peers that "my old man won't let me," it is a convenient "out" for them not to participate in activities that they didn't want to do in the first place. This allows them to save face with their peers.

Most parents of teens want their teen to grow up but often they also want them to remain a child under their influence. Even though teens tend to reject, spurn, and ignore the advice of parents, parents nonetheless must persevere in the challenge to keep the lines of communication open. Even though teens may not want hugs and kisses, they do need to know that their parents care enough about them to persist with concerns. Giving up this fight means giving total control to peers and outside influences. Family values cannot survive in that milieu. Even with repeated shoulder shrugs and "whatevers," parents must continue to steer their teen to appropriate choices and to set limits. Communication between parents and teens is crucial to the eventual emergence of a successful, confident adult. As is evident, the societal expectations and challenges for teens are immense and parental struggles during this stage are equally difficult.

© Edyta Pawlowska, 2009. Used under license from Shutterstock, Inc.

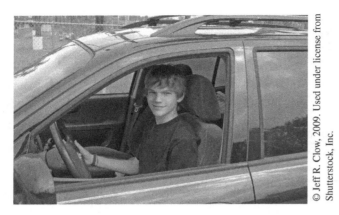

© Jeff R. Clow, 2009. Used under license from Shutterstock, Inc.

Sometime during the teen years, teens are also expected to choose a career path or at least choose a college and a college major. Because they have not had the opportunity to explore so many options, they tend to gravitate to occupations and careers of those they respect. This choice may be to follow in the footsteps of parents or a family friend or associate but is rarely a choice made on a thorough analysis. Rarely are teens aware of the full implications of years of study and years of commitment to a career, so it is not uncommon if they change majors during college

Most teens are also expected to have a job. A job helps make them accountable and responsible. Having a job also helps them to appreciate the value of a dollar and how to save for those "extras" that they want.

Health Concerns

Most of the common teen health issues have already been addressed. These include gender identity, peer pressure, body image, acne, scoliosis, anorexia nervosa, bulimia, exercise-based body dysmorphia, use of steroids, severe depression, teen pregnancy, and sexually transmitted disease. In addition, motor vehicle accidents, the number one cause of death for all ages, is a major concern. Even though teens have the knowledge and physical ability to drive a car, once again their errors in judgment make them especially vulnerable to automobile accidents.

Summary

It certainly is not easy being a teenager in today's world and it certainly is not easy to be a parent of a teenager in today's world. With anticipatory guidance, parents will hopefully be able to meet the challenge to allow the teen to become responsibly independent and self-confident in a very confusing and demanding world.

References

Erikson, E. H. (1968). *Childhood and society* (35th anniversary ed.). New York: Norton.

Kohlberg, L. (1969). *The philosophy of moral development: Vol. 1.* San Francisco: Harper & Row.

Maslow, A. (1968). *Toward a psychology of being* (2nd ed.). New York: Van Nostrand.

Piaget, J. (1950). *The psychology of intelligence.* London: Routledge and Kegan Paul.

Reflection

In the space below, recall one of the most difficult experiences you may have had as a teenager and describe how you were able to resolve it.

Assignment

Complete this form with essential data for Adolescence

Growth and Development Guide for Adolescence

	Physical Traits	Physical Abilities	Psychosocial Task (Erikson)	Evidence of How Achieved	Evidence of Non-Achievement	Cognitive Ability (Piaget)	Evidence of Achievement	Moral Capability (Kohlberg)	Evidence of Achievement
Adolescence 12–18 years									

Name: _____

Study Guide for
Adolescence (12–18 Years)

1. Differentiate the terms: 'Adolescence' and 'Puberty'.

2. Differentiate secondary sex characteristics from primary sex characteristics and describe how and when these appear during the teen years.

   P= Reached Puberty = ability to have a Child

   Secondary = Pubic Hair, Deeping of voice

3. Describe how and why teens so readily confuse sex with dating relationships.

4. Describe the impact of hormones on acne and perspiration during adolescence.

5. Compare and contrast 'peer acceptance' and 'peer pressure'.

6. Describe what it means to have a 'positive' body image.

7. Explain why rebellion and rejection of authority is common during adolescence.

8. Describe what is meant by the 'Fable of Immunity' and give at least one example of how this might be evidenced.

9. Describe the adolescent limitations in cognition relating to choosing options for the future.

10. Explain how limitations in cognition may also affect the moral choices of a teen.

Name: _____

Review

1. A 16 year-old with acne says, "I don't understand why I have it. I stopped eating chocolate, but still have pimples." What should you tell him about the cause of acne?

    a. Acne is caused by pubescent activation of the endocrine gland.

    b. Acne is usually controlled by limiting the excessive intake of fried foods and carbonated beverages.

    c. Acne is related to the excessive outpouring of the hormone estrogen.

    d. Acne is an allergic response to some environmental factor.

2. What is the best descriptor of the fable of immunity that seems to be prevalent during adolescence?

    a. a false belief that they are not vulnerable to communicable disease ✓

    b. a feeling or myth that falsely assures them that bad things won't happen to them ✓

    c. a casual approach to dangerous or evil deeds based on the conviction that if caught, they will not be held responsible since they are under age ✓

    d. the belief that peers will stand by them regardless of circumstances

3. Which of the following are secondary sex characteristics? Choose all that apply.

    a. deepening of the male voice

    b. widening of the female pelvis

    c. female menarche

    d. d. growth of pubic and axillary hair

4. Which of the following best describes body dysmorphia?

    a. experiencing body image misperception and/or distortion

    b. having disproportionate body parts

    c. giving excessive attention to hygiene

    d. wishing one's body to be of a different gender

G&D: ADOLESCENCE

- Ages 12-20
- Physical and Physiologic Characteristics
  - Growth spurt
    - Variances in timing between male / female
    - Anatomical risks
  - Secondary Sex Characteristics
    - Female breast buds, pubic & underarm hair and hip widening
    - Male deepening of voice, pubic, underarm and facial hair

G&D: ADOLESCENCE

- PUBERTY (usually comes first)
  - Physiological changes (hormonal / growth) that occur during pre-teen and teen years
    - Menses (menarche)
    - Wet dreams _males_
    - Glandular secretions: Perspiration, Acne
      - Sexual reproductive ability
        - Craving for love and attention results in confusing this need with sex

G&D: ADOLESCENCE

- Attraction to Opposite Sex
  - Dating
    - Learning self-esteem skills
    - Learning social skills
    - Learning relationship skills
  - Sexual Experimentation
    - Gender Identity Issues
    - Sexually transmitted disease
    - Pregnancy
      - High risk for fetus

Self Esteem skills important.
↳learning about sexuality/Boundaries
Respect,

G&D: ADOLESCENCE

Growth and Physiologic Requirements
- Nutrition: needed for rapid growth but in
  - Fast food world
- Exercise
  - Sports
- Sleep
  - Need 10-12 hours of sleep/night but rarely get

Images used under license from Shutterstock, Inc.

G&D: ADOLESCENCE

Body Image
- Preening in front of mirror excessively
  - How do others perceive me?
    - Body comparisons with peers
  - How do I perceive myself?
    - Body Dysmorphia
      - Eating Disorders F
      - Exercise manias M

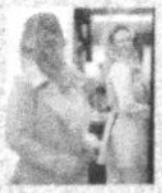

© Yuri Arcurs, 2009

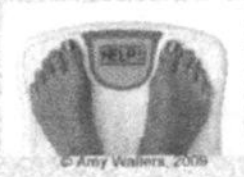

© Amy Walters, 2009

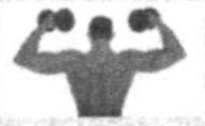

© MaxFX, 2009

Images used under license from Shutterstock, Inc.

Body Dysmorphia - distorted image of self
Bing - Eat / throw up / Anorexia

G&D: ADOLESCENCE

ADOLESCENCE
- Psychological and Emotional maturation
  (some never achieve this)
- Striving for IDENTITY
  - Mood swings
  - Trying on different personalities
  - Peer acceptance vs. Peer pressure
  - Rebellion against authority / parents
    - Rejecting status quo
    - Critical of many things in life
- Sometimes getting lost in Role Confusion

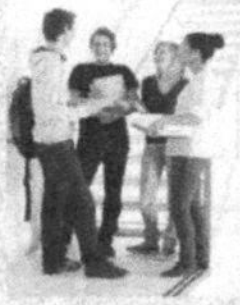

© Yuri Arcurs, 2009.

Images used under license from Shutterstock, Inc.

Puberty = physical changes

Identity

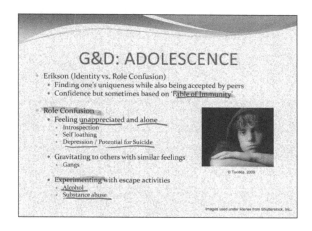

G&D: ADOLESCENCE

Erikson (Identity vs. Role Confusion)
- Finding one's uniqueness while also being accepted by peers
- Confidence but sometimes based on 'Fable of Immunity'

Role Confusion
- Feeling unappreciated and alone
  - Introspection
  - Self loathing
  - Depression / Potential for Suicide
- Gravitating to others with similar feelings
  - Gangs
- Experimenting with escape activities
  - Alcohol
  - Substance abuse

Fable of Immunity – myth nothing Bad
happen to me =

Role confusion = struggle ~~was young ad~~

G&D: ADOLESCENCE

Cognition: Formal Operations (Piaget)
- Can think about thinking
- Introspection
- Can hypothesize about future but lack experience to always make right choices
  - Jobs
  - College
  - Friends

CAN think abstractly.
↳ Deeper thinking / think about future

G&D: ADOLESCENCE

Morality: Social System and Development of Conscience

- Awareness of Societal expectations
- But rejection of Status Quo
- Parental Rules

Think know more than anyone else

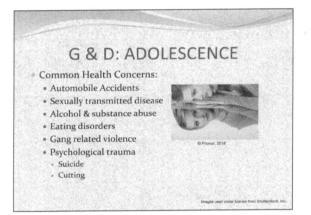

G&D: ADOLESCENCE

* Parental Challenges
  * Rules especially about Independence and Curfews
    * Know that rules will be broken
      * Make consequences to fit crime
      * Make sure consequences are known BEFORE the infraction
    * Teens absolutely hate rules but need rules
      * Safe boundaries
      * Structure
      * Provides choice to obey or not
* Clothes / Hair
* School
* Friends
* Cars

© Jeff R. Clow, 2009

Images used under license from Shutterstock, Inc.

Structure

Setting Boundaries / Setting Rules
Not too strict b/c they need to
'find their way'

G & D: ADOLESCENCE

* Common Health Concerns:
  * Automobile Accidents
  * Sexually transmitted disease
  * Alcohol & substance abuse
  * Eating disorders
  * Gang related violence
  * Psychological trauma
    * Suicide
    * Cutting

© Phovoir, 2018

Images used under license from Shutterstock, Inc.

~~Emergence~~ of Mental health issues

Young Adult (Age 18–35)

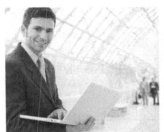

© Zsolt Nyulaszi, 2009. Used under license from Shutterstock, Inc.

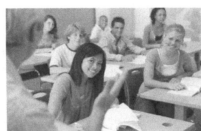

© Monkey Business Images, 2009. Used under license from Shutterstock, Inc.

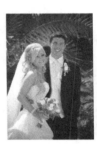

© Karen Grigoryan, 2009. Used under license from Shutterstock, Inc.

Objectives

Upon completion of this chapter, the reader should be able to:

1. Describe the physical characteristics and abilities of the young adult.
2. Give examples of how the psychological task of 'Intimacy' (as described by Erikson) is achieved by young adults.
3. Describe the behaviors associated with 'Isolation' as described by Erikson.
4. Identify risky behaviors that are commonly apparent during young adulthood.
5. Discuss the multiple challenges that are expected to be met during young adulthood.

Key Terms

Fluid Intelligence: speed in cognitive connection and response

Formal Operations: cognition, according to Piaget, that is characterized by the ability to think abstractly, to problem solve with a high level of hypothetical and analytical ability

Intimacy: Erikson's psychosocial task for young adults involving the ability to openly and truly reveal one's inner self to another

Isolation: a sense of aloneness that results from being unsuccessful in achieving Intimacy during young adulthood

Postconventional Morality: behavior, according to Kohlberg, that is based on universal, human principles rather than external regulations

Post-Traumatic Stress Disorder (PTSD): anxiety, depression and a sense of disenfranchisement when trying to reacclimate into society after having experienced a traumatic event

---

Physical Characteristics

The young adult, generally speaking, is in peak physical condition. Growth is complete, the internal organs are at full functional capacity, the joints are at maximum flexibility, and the muscles are fully developed and toned. All physiologic body parts have been developing and building for this climactic moment in time and after this period there will be increasing signs of diminished capacity and function.

Because young adults are so physically fit, they tend to have high energy, stamina, speed, flexibility, strength, endurance, and coordination. The young adult is venturesome and daring and fearless in the face of physical feats that were too risky at a younger age and far too risky for older adults. They will take a dare on a dime. For example, they may attempt rappelling off high cliffs, bungee jumping, sky-diving, skiing, parasailing, and driving race cars. Unintentional injuries secondary to these high-risk behaviors are probably the most common health concern for this age group. Spinal cord injuries result from diving into shallow bodies of water and falls and multiple injuries result from automobile accidents related to speed and/or alcohol.

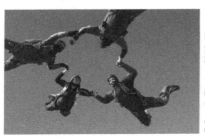
© Joggie Botma, 2009. Used under license from Shutterstock, Inc.

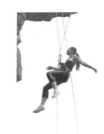
© Zinin Alexei, 2009. Used under license from Shutterstock, Inc.

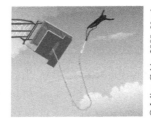
© Jelica Grkic, 2009. Used under license from Shutterstock, Inc.

In addition to taking physical risks that may result in injury, the young adult is also known to engage in activities that may result in disease. Young adults, even though fully aware of the consequences of engaging in unprotected sex, have a high rate of sexually transmitted disease (STD). Even though most sexually transmitted diseases can be treated, there is obvious discomfort in the present and the risk of some long-lasting consequences in the future. HIV can be life threatening, genital warts never go away, and infertility may result from fallopian tube scarring.

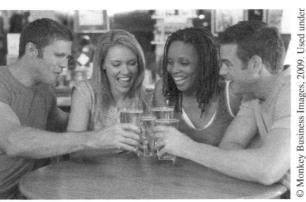
© Monkey Business Images, 2009. Used under license from Shutterstock, Inc.

Young adults also tend to drink alcohol in excess and/or use drugs recreationally. This pattern of behavior, if continued, could cause hepatitis or cirrhosis of the liver in later life. In addition, young adults are frequently found to be driving under the influence of alcohol and or drugs. Smoking cigarettes causes an increased risk of suffering from emphysema or lung cancer.

The high energy peak performance of the young adult is also associated with increased aggression. Young adults, especially the males, do not back down from disputes and often take it to a physical level. Fighting, sometimes involving

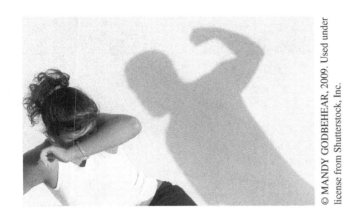

© MANDY GODBEHEAR, 2009. Used under license from Shutterstock, Inc.

lethal weapons like knives and guns, is not uncommon for this age group. Unfortunately, these incidents may result in domestic abuse injuries, homicide, and/or suicide.

Unfortunately, it has also been young adults who have been involved in violent, destructive behaviors in recent years. The bombing at the Boston Marathon and the shootings at the Columbine movie theater and at several schools over the last few years have all been done by young adults.

Health Maintenance Requirements

To sustain the high metabolic rate and energy level of the young adult, optimal nutrition is required. But because young adults are always on the go, they tend to eat on the run and/or eat convenient fast foods. Nutritional deficits are apparent in some young adults who may not have overcome their distorted body image issues and continue in the cycle of eating disorders. There is also an increasing number of obese young adults.

The young adult also requires 6 to 8 hours of sleep each night, but this too is usually not a priority and usually is deficient. Young adults also need physical exercise to sustain their muscle tone and to increase their cardiopulmonary capacity. Hypertension, some genetically based and some stress induced, is commonly diagnosed during the young adult years.

Young adults are the most likely age group not to have health insurance. Under the Patient Protection and Affordable Care Act (2010), young adults could be carried on their parents' policies up to age 26 if they remained in school. But working young adults (especially those who were not offered employer coverage) were forced to pay extremely high premiums for their own policies. Now that the mandate for health insurance is no longer viable, young adults will most likely choose not to be insured because they consider themselves healthy. Furthermore, because they generally feel so good, they tend not to go to the doctor for regular checkups. This may result in untreated or late treated conditions that have poor prognoses. A major health concern for the young adult is cancer. Young adult males are at a prime age for testicular cancer and young adult females are at a prime age for ovarian and cervical cancer. With or without insurance, young adults are highly encouraged to be alert to symptoms and to obtain routine checkups. Early identification and treatment are obviously the best way to have a favorable prognosis.

Societal Expectations

The young adult faces many societal expectations. They need to learn a trade or go to college and earn a degree, serve in the military, get a job and establish a career, and get married and start a family.

Young adults are expected to pay their own way and to live on their own. In order to do that, they must have a job. Many young adults may have already attained job experience during their teen years. This experience may pave the way or give them skills that they can use so they can obtain full-time employment. Other young adults may obtain marketable skills through a trade or business school. Either of these scenarios puts the young adult into the work world relatively quickly.

But getting a higher paying job in today's business world very often requires that one have a college degree. To earn that degree, most young adults spend 4 to 8 years of their life and have to work in order to pay for tuition or take out student loans that may leave them financially strained for many years to come. College can be even more stressful if the young adult has family responsibilities.

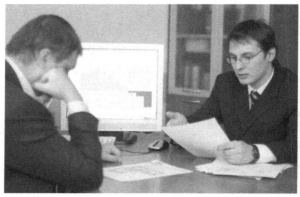
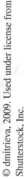

Other young adults are recruited to serve in the military. While the military offers education, travel, salary, and health care, the expectations for frequent relocation and rigorous physical protocols including the possibility of active combat are immense. The military is an especially difficult lifestyle for those young adults with family responsibilities. And there is a growing major concern related to Post-Traumatic Stress Disorder (PTSD). Many who have served our country well in combat, have an extremely difficult time re-adjusting to the every-day comforts of U.S. society.

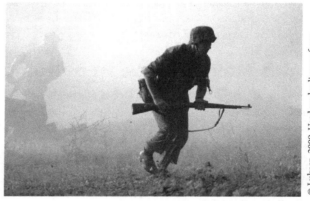

And then to top off these high demands, the young adult is expected to settle down, get married, and start a family. This sequencing of life choices is the ideal. As indicated above, very often, being married and having children all too often precedes getting a job or earning a degree or serving in the military. This, of course, complicates the entire scene.

Because the physical condition of the young adult is optimal, this is also a prime time for pregnancy. The young adult female body is well suited for child bearing and for bearing healthy babies. The ovaries have a limited supply of eggs to be fertilized and the older the female becomes, the less likely that the eggs will be healthy and viable. As stated above, nutrition for the young adult is not always optimal and for the pregnant young adult this is a major concern. The young adult is also well suited to child rearing. During this time of life when young adults have a high level of energy, they are more able and apt to keep up with the high energy demands of taking care of infants and toddlers.

If married and optimally prepared, pregnancy and the birth of a child are beautiful blessings. But pregnancy, for the young adult, is not always a welcome event. Even though they are a bit older and wiser, unplanned pregnancies can and do occur. Sometimes this means putting an up-and-coming career on hold or carries a financial burden that the young adult is not prepared for. This can be a very stressful situation.

Developmental Theories

Intimacy vs. Isolation (Erikson)

According to Erikson (1969), the young adult is expected to achieve the task of **intimacy**. Intimacy has very little to do with sexual relations but it may include sexual relations as part of the bigger picture. Intimacy means revealing one's inner self, one's private self, and sharing this with another. Intimacy requires self-disclosure of

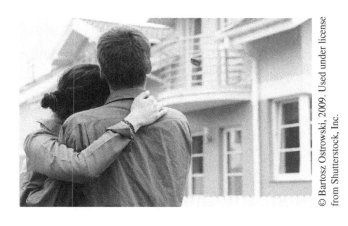

the "real me" without pretense or barriers. Intimacy requires a strong sense of mutual trust that, when sharing deeply held feelings, one will be understood, will still be accepted, and will still be loved.

Intimacy requires truly loving another without having selfish hidden agendas. Intimacy also requires an individual to allow this special other person to love them just the way they are. This is what marriage is intended to be, two persons knowing and loving each other in the deepest sense of the word. It follows that this unity of mind is further enhanced when there is sexual union as well. Intimacy may be accomplished with members of the same sex as well as with members of the opposite sex. The same principles apply. What is most essential in finding a life partner is the psychosocial connection and commitment. The legalization of same sex marriages has made this connection and commitment a reality for many.

But finding true intimacy is a very difficult task for many. Finding that special someone, a soul mate, someone with whom one can share their most intimate thoughts, is not easy. Often dating individuals find themselves caught up in the physical attraction and the soul mate perspective gets overshadowed.

There are many young adults who may never find or who may choose not to seek a life partner. So can these individuals achieve intimacy? Yes. They can successfully achieve the task of intimacy through a commitment to their work or to a cause. Their passion and deep feelings about this involvement are quite sufficient to allow them to feel complete.

Young adults who are not successful in achieving intimacy tend to isolate themselves from the rest of the world. It is possible that they feel themselves to be a failure and fear further rejection or failure. These individuals tend to avoid involvement and participation in social events and rarely commit to their work. This stage of **isolation** is evident in their unhappy demeanor. They tend to be critical of and mad at the world. As indicated previously, isolation is also a growing concern for returning members of the military who are experiencing Post-Traumatic Stress Disorder (PTSD).

Many individuals who are experiencing isolation become deeply depressed. This is apparent in their posture (slouching and slumping), their gait (slow and dragging), speech (monotone without interest), insomnia (inability to sleep), and gastrointestinal disorders (vomiting and diarrhea). These individuals obviously need professional counseling and medication. The pressures to get a degree, get a job, get settled, get married, and start a family are sometimes overwhelming to the young adult. Unfortunately, suicide is a major concern for this age group and must be guarded against. Young adult females actually attempt suicide more frequently but it is the young adult males who are the most successful in completion of the deed.

Cognition: Formal Operations (Piaget)

According to Piaget (1950), young adults are at a peak in formal operations cognition. They are quick witted, have an amazing speed of recall, speed in cognitive connections and responses and can quickly analyze and solve problems. This is known as having **fluid intelligence**. For this reason, many young adults are extremely successful in launching their careers.

Young adults are more perceptive, insightful, and analytical than adolescents. They are able to more objectively and realistically evaluate issues as well as to construct hypotheses and test them analytically. They are also more rational in making social and occupational decisions and commitments like marriage and career, and in establishing financial and residential independence.

Because young adults are young and daring and lack experience, they sometimes err in taking a chance. But because they are young and daring, they tend to bounce back quickly. Since they don't have years and years of time invested or life savings invested, they have plenty of time to re-group and try again. It is a wonderful time of life to take these risks.

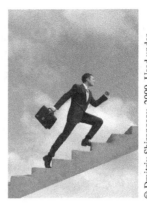

© Dmitriy Shironosov, 2009. Used under license from Shutterstock, Inc.

Morality: Postconventional (Kohlberg)

According to Kohlberg (1969), young adults are capable of **postconventional morality**. Postconventional morality is characterized by actions that are based on principles rather than on external regulations.

Individuals with postconventional morality have an internal ethic that is demonstrated in respect and care for others. These individuals may stop on busy streets to allow cars on the side streets to move into traffic. They do this not because it is law, but because it is the right thing to do. They donate money to charity because they want to, not because they have to.

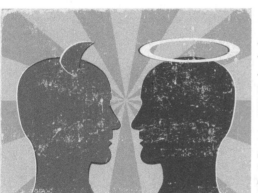

© Portia Remnant, 2009. Used under license from Shutterstock, Inc.

Even though young adults have the capability of demonstrating postconventional behaviors, this does not mean that they always and only perform in this realm. It is not uncommon for many young adults to occasionally behave at lower levels of moral aptitude. Many young adults have, on some occasion, done something good only in order to gain something in return (instrumental purpose and exchange). Many young adults also follow rules just because they are rules (conventional) or because they fear the repercussions (fear and punishment). Behaviors of this sort are obviously not restricted to young adults. Adults of all ages behave similarly. According to Kohlberg's theory of morality, it is very normal for most people to fluctuate in morality, based on the motive of the moment.

Summary

Young adulthood is an exciting and productive time of life. It is also a time of immense pressure related to societal expectations. Thankfully, most young adults achieve intimacy and flourish in their fluid intelligence and make great contributions to the world.

References

Erikson, E. H. (1968). *Childhood and society* (35th anniversary ed.). New York: Norton.
Healthcare: Patient Protection and Affordable Health Care Act 2010 (Retrieved from healthcare.gov 5/30/2015)
Kohlberg, L. (1969). *The philosophy of moral development: Vol. 1*. San Francisco: Harper & Row.
Piaget, J. (1950). *The psychology of intelligence*. London: Routledge and Kegan Paul.

Reflection

In the space below, recall and describe a societal expectation that was difficult for you during young adulthood

Assignment

Complete this form with essential data for the Young Adult

Growth and Development Guide for the Young Adult

	Physical Traits	Physical Abilities	Psychosocial Task (Erikson)	Evidence of How Achieved	Evidence of Non-Achievement	Cognitive Ability (Piaget)	Evidence of Achievement	Moral Capability (Kohlberg)	Evidence of Achievement
Young Adult (18–35 years)									

Name: _____

Study Guide for
Young Adult (18–35 Years)

1. Explain what it means for the Young Adult to be in 'peak' physical condition.

2. Describe how the peak physical condition of the Young Adult may lead to risky behavior and inadvertent injury.

3. Describe the societal expectations that are often imposed on the Young Adult.

4. Differentiate 'Intimacy' as described by Erikson from sexual intimacy.

5. Explain how commitment to a career or cause fulfills the task of 'Intimacy'.

6. Compare and contrast the formal operations capability of the Young Adult to that of an Adolescent.

7. Explain the pros and cons of undertaking business and financial risks during Young Adulthood.

8. Describe what is meant by 'fluid intelligence' and how this is evidenced during the Young Adult years.

9. Explain what is meant by 'postconventional' morality according to Kohlberg.

10. Explain how and why individuals do not always act from the moral perspective that has been identified as appropriate to their age.

Name: _____

Review

1. Which of the following best describes fluid intelligence?

    a. wisdom in seeing the big picture
    b. ability to perform detailed analyses of problems
    (c.) speed in cognitive connections and responses
    d. deductive reasoning

2. Why are unintentional injuries a common cause of death among young adults?

    (a.) Because young adults feel so healthy and alive, they are prone to engage in risky and/or dangerous behaviors.
    b. Young adults are so busy in seeking careers and partners that they don't take time to think about their actions.
    c. Young adults strive to succeed but do not yet have all the coping skills to accomplish goals.
    d. Young adults do not yet have the ability to realize the consequences of their actions.

3. Which of the following best describes 'Intimacy' as explained by Erikson?

    a. Positioning one's self in very close proximity to another
    (b.) Revealing one's inner self to another
    c. Having sexual relations with another
    d. Sharing information with another

4. Which of the following situations is most likely to lead to young adult "Isolation?" Choose all that apply.

    (a.) being rejected by a lover ✓
    b. being highly committed to a cause ✗
    (c.) non-participation in societal events ✓
    d. being overly committed to a successful career ✗

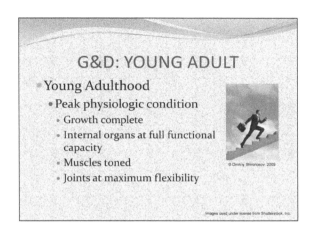

G&D: YOUNG ADULT

- Young Adulthood
  - Peak physiologic condition
    - Growth complete
    - Internal organs at full functional capacity
    - Muscles toned
    - Joints at maximum flexibility

© Dmitry Shironosov, 2009

Images used under license from Shutterstock, Inc.

G&D: YOUNG ADULT

- Risky behaviors associated with **high energy, stamina,** speed, flexibility, strength endurance and coordination;
- Physically dangerous stunts
  - ⟶ spinal cord injuries
- Failure to use protection in sexual encounters
  - ⟶ STDs and unwanted pregnancies
- Driving under the influence of alcohol or drugs
  - ⟶ injury to self or others

© Monkey Business Images, 2009

Images used under license from Shutterstock, Inc.

PRONE to Risky Behaviors.

G&D: YOUNG ADULT

- Injuries especially traumatic for Young Adult related to
  - Full future ahead of them
    - Finishing College
    - Starting Career
    - Beginning Family
  - Spinal injuries especially devastating and financially draining

© Zhan Alexei, 2009

Images used under license from Shutterstock, Inc.

Abstract / formal thinking / cognition.

G&D: YOUNG ADULT

Aggression
- Especially associated with young adult males
  - Fist fights at bars
  - Domestic abuse
  - Gun / knife injuries
  - Road rage
  - Violent destructive behaviors
    - Taking innocent lives

↑ homicide

G&D: YOUNG ADULT

- Health Maintenance Requirements
  - Optimal nutrition but in fast food 'convenience' world
  - Routine exercise necessary
  - Need 6-8 hours of sleep/night
  - Infrequent consumers of recommended screenings (PAP smear)(Testicular)
  - Diseases become advanced and more difficult to treat

Still thinking "nothing will happen to me"

Screening for Depression (mental Health)

G&D: YOUNG ADULT

Social Expectations
- Education
- Job
- Live on own and pay own bills
- Get married
- Start a family
- Buy a house
- Enlist in Military

G&D: YOUNG ADULT

- Pregnancy during Young Adult years
  - Delight
    - Optimal physical condition
    - Planned and wanted child

  - Maybe not
    - Increased responsibility and bills

© Lana K, 2009

Images used under license from Shutterstock, Inc.

G&D: YOUNG ADULT

- Psychosocial Task: <u>INTIMACY</u> (Erikson)   v. Isolation
  - Feeling comfortable with who I am
  - Feeling comfortable with being by self with strong friend support system
  - Feeling comfortable to share those innermost feelings with another individual
    - Trust
    - Acceptance
    - Love and being loved

© Karen Grigoryan, 2009

Images used under license from Shutterstock, Inc.

having passion for a cause.

G&D: YOUNG ADULT

- ISOLATION
  - Feeling of failure in achieving societal expectations
  - Feeling of rejection in interpersonal relationships

    - DEPRESSION
      - Inactivity; lack of productivity
      - Absence of social contacts
      - Potential for sad introspection resulting in suicide

© Bruna Ray, 2009

Images used under license from Shutterstock, Inc.

G&D: YOUNG ADULT

COGNITION: Formal Operations (Piaget)
- Fluid intelligence at peak performance
  level but tend to lack experience
- Willing to take chances because
  they have less to lose, and
  they have time to pick up and start again

© Zsolt Nyulaszi, 2009.

MORALITY: Post-Conventional Ability
but not always acting at that level
↳ change possible

© Bananaboy, 2016

Images used under license from Shutterstock, Inc.

Not concrete.

Middle-Age (35–65)

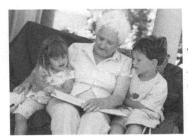

© Monkey Business Images, 2009. Used under license from Shutterstock, Inc.

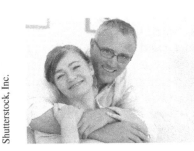

© Yuri Arcurs, 2009. Used under license from Shutterstock, Inc.

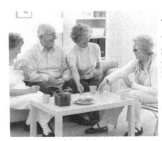

© Yuri Arcurs, 2009. Used under license from Shutterstock, Inc.

Objectives

Upon completion of this chapter, the reader should be able to:

1. Describe the physical and physiological changes associated with middle age.
2. Describe the nutritional and exercise recommendations appropriate for the middle-aged adult.
3. Describe common chronic conditions that tend to appear during middle age.
4. Explain "generativity" as described by Erikson as the psychosocial task for middle-aged adults.
5. Describe the role of work and effective use of leisure as related to accomplishing generativity.
6. Explain "stagnation" as described by Erikson as the absence of "generativity."
7. Compare and contrast "fluid intelligence" and "crystallized intelligence."

Key Terms

Crystallized intelligence: wisdom (derived from accumulated knowledge and life experiences) in personal choices and in advice to others

Fluid intelligence: speed in cognitive connections and responses; having the ability to quickly analyze situations and respond appropriately

Generativity: the psychosocial task of middle age, according to Erikson, that is characterized by a willingness to share knowledge and experience with the younger generations

Launching: preparing adult children to live and function independently

Middle-age spread: the tendency to gain weight especially around the waist that occurs during middle age as a result of decreased metabolism and decreased exercise coupled with less than optimal nutrition

Presbycusis: loss of hearing related to the loss of fluid lubrication for the middle ear bones of conduction

Presbyopia: loss of nearsightedness commonly occurring during middle age

Stagnation: a psychosocial perspective of indifference to others and increased focus on one's own needs

---

Physical and Physiological Characteristics

There are multiple physical and physiological changes that occur during middle age and most of these changes are degenerative, that is, evidencing loss of previously held characteristics. Hair becomes thinner, loses its pigment, and turns gray. The pubic and underarm hair also thins and becomes sparse. There is a decrease in subcutaneous tissue, causing the skin to lose its elasticity and making wrinkles more apparent. The skin also undergoes some pigment changes resulting in age spots, especially in areas previously exposed to the sun like on the face and arms.

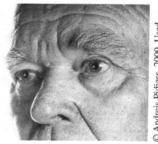

© Andrejs Pidjass, 2009. Used under license from Shutterstock, Inc.

There is also a change in the shape of the eye causing the middle-aged adult to lose some peripheral vision which makes driving somewhat hazardous. And most middle age adults need bifocal lenses or reading glasses to read small print. This loss of nearsightedness is called **presbyopia**. Other vision-related conditions sometimes seen in middle-aged adults, include glaucoma and cataracts.

There may also be some loss of hearing related to the decreased lubrication of the bones of the middle ear resulting in decreased conduction of sound. This is known as **presbycusis**. There is some decrease in taste and smell as well, but these are not generally as pronounced. One of the more common changes in taste relates to salt. Because salt flavoring is not readily sensed in middle-aged adults, they tend to add excessive table salt to their foods. This is turn causes fluid retention and potentiates hypertension and other cardiopulmonary problems.

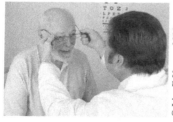

© Lisa F. Young, 2009. Used under license from Shutterstock, Inc.

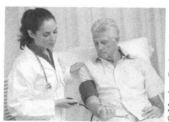

© Monkey Business Images, 2009. Used under license from Shutterstock, Inc.

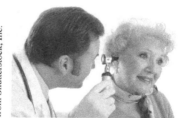

© Lisa F. Young, 2009. Used under license from Shutterstock, Inc.

In general, there is less fluid in the body during middle age. This is apparent in decreased flexibility in the joints. With the loss of fluid plus the normal wear and tear of joints, there may be stiffness and/or bone-on-bone creaking with joint movement. If the body is deficient in calcium, the long bones will readily release calcium causing an increased bone fragility and increased risk for falls and fractures. The vertebrae in the spinal column also lose some fluid cushioning. This again results in decreased flexibility and often results in the middle-aged person shrinking somewhat in height.

Did you know?

Did you know that many of the type 2 diabetes cases that are diagnosed during middle age is related to increased weight gain? Are you aware of the connection between fat cells and cellular resistance to insulin?

There may also be an increase in weight. The **middle-age spread** is a phenomenon that results primarily from a physiologic shift in metabolism. When decreased metabolism is coupled with poor nutrition and minimal exercise, there is inevitably an increase in weight. Middle-aged adults are certainly encouraged to decrease their caloric intake, but very often, many continue to eat in a manner similar to when they were in their young adult years. The decreased metabolism means that weight can be gained much more readily and losing weight will take a lot longer.

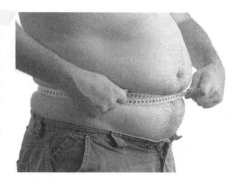

© Ljupco Smokovski, 2009. Used under license from Shutterstock, Inc.

Health Maintenance

The middle-aged adult needs to exercise. They need aerobic exercise to maintain heart and lung health, but they may need longer periods of warm-up and cool-down to minimize the risk for excessive strain or pull. They also need physical exercise to maximize mobility and flexibility and to release the endorphins that make them feel better all over. Middle-aged adults also need resistance (anaerobic) exercises to maximize joint mobility and flexibility. Exercise for the middle-aged adult should be moderate but consistently maintained in practice. A minimum exercise regimen of 3 to 5 times a week is highly recommended.

One of the best exercises for the middle-aged adult is walking. Walking increases heart and lung capacity, stimulates the circulation, improves the kinesthetic sense of balance, increases muscle tone, and strengthens the long bones. All middle-aged adults should be highly encouraged to walk 6 to 8 miles/week. Swimming is also an excellent exercise for middle-aged adults because of the absence of pressure on the weight-bearing joints. Of course, most middle-aged adults are quite capable of engaging in other more physical activities like tennis or golf but they just need to listen to the limits of their bodies. Absence of exercise will result in decreased stability and reduced mobility.

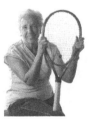

© Carme Balcells, 2009. Used under license from Shutterstock, Inc.

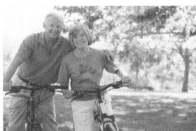

© Monkey Business Images, 2009. Used under license from Shutterstock, Inc.

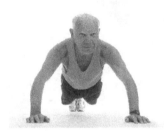

© Glenda M. Powers, 2009. Used under license from Shutterstock, Inc.

Hormonal Changes

There also are hormonal changes that occur during middle age years. Females commonly experience symptoms of pre-menopause and menopause in their 40s and 50s. A shift in the hormonal levels of estrogen is primarily responsible for the common symptoms of hot flashes and mood swings. When menopause is complete, the release of estrogen is essentially nonexistent. Because estrogen is protective of the calcium in the bones, women are at a greater risk for long bone fragility after

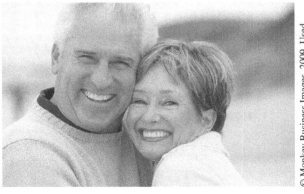

© Monkey Business Images, 2009. Used under license from Shutterstock, Inc.

menopause. Some women may need a hormonal estrogen supplement to transition through the symptoms and/or to stabilize the calcium levels. Following menopause, females are no longer able to conceive and bear children. This in no way implies that they lose their sexual libido. It is not uncommon for middle-aged women to desire and enjoy sexual activities even more because they do not have the worry of unplanned pregnancy.

Related to the loss of muscle tone in the abdominal area as a result of repeated pregnancies and deliveries, many middle-aged females experience increased pressure on the bladder and/or gravitational pull of the uterus. Incontinence and/or severe abdominal discomfort may require surgical intervention (hysterectomy, oopherectomy, and bladder suspension).

There is also a loss of hormonal secretion in males. Even though this does not in any way diminish the male capacity to father a child, or in their libido, there may be some mood swings and in some cases, a diminished capacity to obtain and sustain an erection. This is usually treated with medications (the famous little 'blue' pill). Men sometimes experience a "mid-life crisis," a perception of themselves as less virile than in earlier years. Stereotypical behaviors for men in mid-life crisis include compensatory actions like dyeing their hair or changing their hair style, buying a sports car or boat, or flirting with a younger woman.

Another common hormonally related problem for males is related to the prostate gland. Benign prostatic hypertrophy (BPH) is a condition in which the prostate gland swells and occludes the passage of urine through the urethra. This can usually be treated effectively with medications that will minimize the swelling in the prostate or with resection surgery that bypasses the occlusion. Prostatic cancer causes similar symptoms but obviously requires surgical and/or chemotherapy and/or radiation intervention.

Chronic Illness

It is not uncommon for individuals in their middle years to experience some chronic diseases or conditions. This does not mean that these conditions or diseases just happen during this time, but that they become apparent during this time. Type 2 diabetes mellitus may become apparent because of the decreased metabolism and the possibility of less than optimal nutrition and/or increased weight. This in turn may result in increased cellular resistance to insulin.

Arthritis may become apparent related to the decreased mobility and flexibility of the joints. Peripheral vascular disease may become apparent related to decreased exercise and the resultant limitations in circulation. Coronary heart disease, atherosclerosis, and/or hypertension may be genetically linked or related to years and years of stress, but may also be related to dietary deficits and insufficient exercise.

Most chronic conditions that tend to surface during middle age are a result of behavioral and/or dietary deficits that have been carried over from younger years. These include poor nutrition, lack of exercise, periodontal disease, alcoholism (cir-

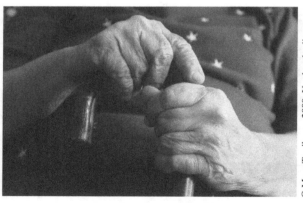
© Mary Terriberry, 2009. Used under license from Shutterstock, Inc.

rhosis), and lung cancer and/or emphysema (related to smoking). With a decrease in metabolism and in immune response, the middle-aged individual is more likely to show symptoms of these problems than in earlier years.

The 'Golden Years'

In spite of all of the deteriorating body parts and declining function, the middle age years are often referred to as the "golden years." This is because it is a time when most individuals experience a high level of self-satisfaction in their lives. The middle-aged adult generally has a firm grasp of expertise in their career, has sufficient financial stability to live comfortably, and has successfully "launched" their children to function on their own. In other words, the pressures of earlier years, for the most part, are now minimized.

A challenge for middle-aged adults is to successfully launch their own children out into the world. **Launching** means preparing their children to live independently and on their own and then comfortably "cutting those apron strings." This may involve supporting them through college or while learning a skill set for employment. Or it may mean supporting them in their early marriage and child-bearing years by providing some babysitting services and/or financial assistance until they can function on their own. It almost always means encouraging their children to move out of the house and to provide their own meals and laundry services.

Many times after launching has occurred, middle-aged adults have to reestablish a life with their spouse or life partner. Oftentimes, there may have been such demand for attention given to the children that the marital relationship may have suffered. After launching, the couples need to relearn how to live and love their partners. Sometimes, this is not a happy rediscovery and could lead to separation and/or divorce. The loneliness and uncertainties of life that ensue frequently cause severe depression in one or both spouses. Dating and/or re-marrying at this age could be fun and/or exciting but it could also be very scary and undesirable.

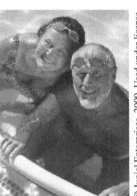

© Junial Enterprises, 2009. Used under license from Shutterstock, Inc.

The same situation could happen if one of the spouses becomes ill and/or dies. There is increased demand on the healthy spouse and a definite decline in the enjoyment that they were supposed to have at this stage in their lives.

One of the greatest concerns for the middle-aged adult is related to preparing for retirement. One cannot just decide to retire from a lifelong career without careful planning. One simply cannot stop a routine that has become an integral part of their life for many years without having some consequences. The middle-aged adult needs to stay involved in some productive activity, with or without a paying job.

Retirement should never be cessation of activity but rather a conscious choice of activities that have been deferred because of lack of time or availability. This may be in activities that bring them relaxation pleasure. Many retirees take time to travel around the world, while others may find total contentment in spending time with their grand-children. Others volunteer their service at churches or schools or hospitals and others take up gardening or knitting or baking. Many retired middle-aged individuals go back to school to learn something they always wanted to know and take up a new and exciting hobby. In all situations, they are continuing to be productive and feel good about what they are doing rather than being obligated to do these things. This may also mean that they could continue to serve as consultants in their former workplace.

Did you know?

Did you know that since many middle-aged individuals define themselves by their job and/or career, they tend to have minimal outside interests and therefore do not know how to relax and enjoy life. These individuals have a much more difficult time in letting go of work and finding meaning in other activities. Retirement, for them, is NOT welcomed or an anticipated event.

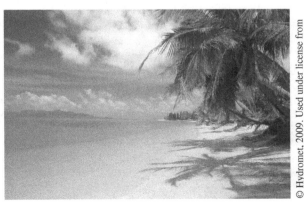

© Hydromet, 2009. Used under license from Shutterstock, Inc.

Developmental Theories

Generativity vs. Stagnation (Erikson)

Middle-aged adults need to feel needed and they have a lot to ooffer. According to Erikson (1969), the middle-aged adult needs to accomplish **generativity**. Generativity is characterized by activities that evidence a desire and willingness to share with the younger generations, their wisdom and expertise in multiple areas. Most middle-aged adults have become experts in their career fields and are looked up to for insight and perspective. The middle-aged adult is highly respected in family circles and is proud to share their life experiences in order to help others to cope with current issues. Reviewing their past accomplishments makes most middle-aged adults feel very successful and good about themselves.

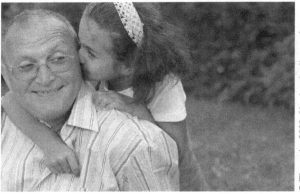

© Timurpix, 2009. Used under license from Shutterstock, Inc.

There is a risk that introspection could result in depression because they have not been as successful as they wished they had been or had as much money as they wanted to have or owned some things that they always wanted. This is unhealthy and may cause the middle-aged adult to become stagnant.

Stagnation, the opposing psychosocial characteristic for middle-aged adults, implies that they are doing nothing, and are contributing nothing to the betterment

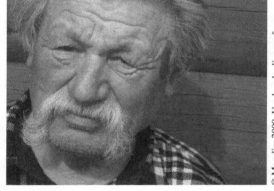

© Marylin, 2009. Used under license from Shutterstock, Inc.

of the world. Middle-aged persons in stagnation often become preoccupied with their own health and/or wealth and want to keep totally to themselves and shun social interaction with others. Middle-aged individuals in stagnation, are consumed with their own idleness and tend to be very unhappy individuals.

Cognition: Formal Operations/Crystallized Intelligence (Piaget)

Generativity is closely linked with formal operations, as described by Piaget (1950). As has been described about the declining body parts in middle age, the neural connections for thought processing also become somewhat compromised. This does not mean that middle-aged adults are less intelligent but it does mean that their intelligence is in their wisdom rather than in speed of recall. A middle-aged adult has **crystallized intelligence**, an accumulation of knowledge and experience that makes them very wise in their choices and in the advice that they give. But with increased age there may be some decrease in **fluid intelligence**. This means that they may need a bit more time to remember names or dates, but they will remember. It just takes longer for the processing to take place.

Morality: Postconventional Universal Ethical Principles (Kohlberg)

According to Kohlberg, the middle age adult is capable of acting on principals rather than for rewards, acknowledgements or societal expectations. For example, middle age adults are likely to stop and help someone who has fallen or who has dropped something. Universal ethical principals dictate that individuals do what is inherently right, that is, they know that this is the right thing to do and they do it. If they find something of value, they are likely to return it to the rightful owner. But as indicated in each of the age groups, Kohlberg readily admits that even though the middle age adult has this capability, this does not mean that they always act in this realm. Reverting back to a previous stage of morality can and does occur.

Summary

Middle Age is a 'golden' time. The kids are raised and on their own, finances are stabilizing and retirement is generally a welcome option. Travel, volunteering, and enjoying the grandchildren make middle age a delightful time of life IF chronic disease does not interfere.

References

Erikson, E. H. (1968). *Childhood and society* (35th anniversary ed.). New York: Norton.

Kohlberg, L. (1969). *The philosophy of moral development: Vol. 1*. San Francisco: Harper & Row.

Piaget, J. (1950). *The psychology of intelligence*. London: Routledge and Kegan Paul.

Reflection

In the space below, think about someone you know in this middle age group and describe how they match (or don't match) the theory as explained in this chapter.

Assignment

Complete this form with essential data for Middle Age

Growth and Development Guide for Middle Age

	Physical Traits	Physical Abilities	Psychosocial Task (Erikson)	Evidence of How Achieved	Evidence of Non-Achievement	Cognitive Ability (Piaget)	Evidence of Achievement	Moral Capability (Kohlberg)	Evidence of Achievement
Middle Age (35–65 years)									

Name: _____

Study Guide for Middle Age (35–65 Years)

1. Explain why the caloric requirement for Middle Age adults is substantially decreased from that which was required during Young Adulthood.

2. Explain why wrinkles tend to become apparent during Middle Age.

3. Explain why Middle Age adults tend to need 'reading' glasses.

4. Explain why Middle Age adults tend to have a 'middle age spread'.

5. Describe the impact of hormonal changes for both males and females during their Middle Age years.

6. Explain how and why chronic diseases tend to be more apparent in Middle Age than ever before.

7. Specify at least three ways in which a Middle Age adult would demonstrate 'Generativity'.

8. Explain why it is important for the Middle Age adult to PLAN for retirement.

9. Describe how and why fluid intelligence and crystallized intelligence both contribute to career expertise during Middle Age.

10. Describe what is meant by Universal Ethical Principles and how it applies to the Middle Age adult.

Name: _____

Review

1. Which of the following statements about middle adulthood is <u>not</u> true?

   a. Females usually experience a decrease in the enjoyment of sexual activity. ✗
   b. Males maintain the capability of reproduction throughout their adult lives. ✓
   c. Males frequently experience emotional crisis during middle adulthood years. ✓
   d. Menopause ends the possibility of future reproduction for females. ✓

2. Which of the following is the greatest contributor to the appearance of chronic disease in the middle-aged adult?

   a. decreased energy to seek medical attention
   b. acute illness related to decreased immune response
   c. psychological depression related to aging
   d. unhealthy earlier lifestyles

3. Which of the following best describes 'launching'?

   a. taking time to travel
   b. breaking away from a career
   c. untying the apron strings and letting children establish their own lives
   d. taking on a new hobby

4. When middle age Mrs. Jones states: "I've been working and doing things for others most of my life; now it is 'me' time and time to do nothing", she is expressing…..

   a. generativity ✗
   b. universal ethical principals ✗
   c. body dysmorphia ✗
   d. stagnation ✗

Prenatal development.

Human Cognitive development - Piaget.

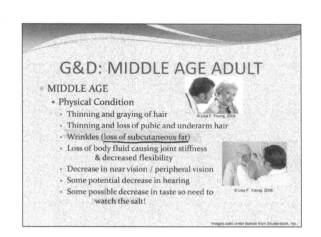

Important to drink H2O

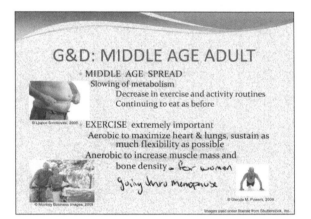

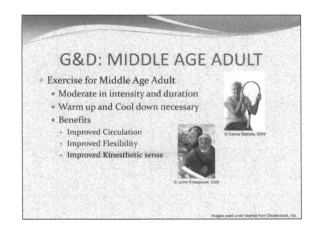

Kinesthetic Space = aware of Body, Space
- Balance

G&D: MIDDLE AGE ADULT

- Hormonal Changes
  - Female Menopause Late 40s - 50s
    - Loss of estrogen=loss of ability to sustain calcium in long bones=tendency for osteoporosis
  - Male Mid-Life Crisis
  - No physiologic reason for loss of libido

- Common Physiologic Changes
  - Female bladder control issues
  - Male prostatic enlargement

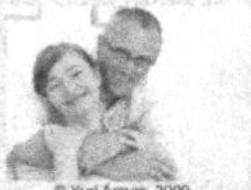

© Yuri Arcurs, 2009

Images used under license from Shutterstock, Inc.

Stop menstrating = loss of estrogen
calcium - no longer protected by estrogen
↳ means more prone for osteoprerosis

G&D: MIDDLE AGE ADULT

- Health Concerns
  - Chronic Diseases 40s-60s
    - Causes
      - Genetics
      - Lifestyle behaviors
    - Diabetes Mellitus
    - Arthritis
    - Coronary Heart Disease
    - Hypertension
    - Emphysema ~~long~~ Smokers
    - Alcoholism - Liver Failure

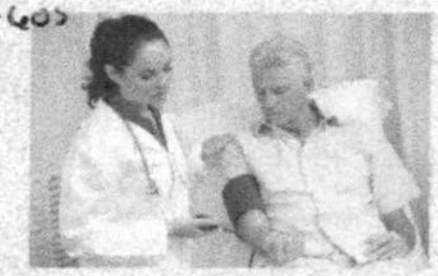

© Monkey Business Images, 2009

Images used under license from Shutterstock, Inc.

Genetic Predispositions does not mean you will get it

G&D: MIDDLE AGE ADULT

- Golden Years
  - Expertise in Career
  - Financially stable
  - Children launched into lives of their own
  - More time to self
  - Time to re-establish personal relationship with spouse
  - Retirement potential

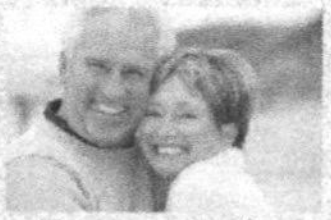

© Monkey Business Images, 2009

Images used under license from Shutterstock, Inc.

Grown in wisedom-/ Experience

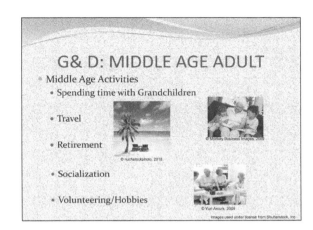

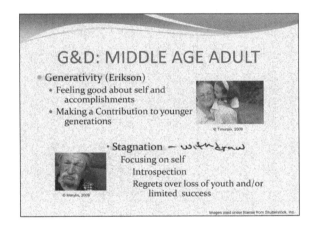

Generativity = feels good sharing
move forward w/ life

Stagnation - Regrets on things did not do

G&D: MIDDLE AGE ADULT

COGNITION: Formal Operations
- Fluid Intelligence
  - Some decrease in speed but
  - Expertise
  - Experience
- Crystallized Intelligence
  - Wisdom
    - Many years of experience allows better choices because of awareness of consequences
  - Able to see big picture

Fluid Intellegence - can recall quickly
Crystal Intelligence - "wisdom"
↳ learning on own.

G&D: MIDDLE AGE ADULT

- Morality: Universal Ethical Principals

- Doing the right thing for the right reason

- Because it IS the right thing to do

The Older Adult (Age 65+)

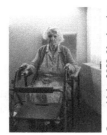

© max blain, 2009. Used under license from Shutterstock, Inc.

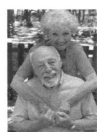

© Lisa F. Young, 2009. Used under license from Shutterstock, Inc.

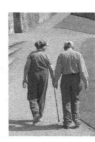

© marylin barbone, 2009. Used under license from Shutterstock, Inc.

Objectives

Upon completion of this chapter, the reader should be able to:

1. Describe the physical and physiological changes commonly found in the older adult.
2. Relate increased longevity to the increased risk for multiple chronic conditions and polypharmacy.
3. Discuss the benefits and limitations of Medicare for the elderly.
4. Explain "Integrity" as described by Erikson as the task to be achieved by the elder individual.
5. Discuss the need for reminiscing and socialization in the elder years.
6. Differentiate Alzheimer's disease and minor memory loss.
7. Describe elder abuse and associated risks.

Key Terms

Activities of Daily Living (ADL): the everyday self-care activities relating to eating, toileting, hygiene, dressing, transfer, and mobility

Alzheimer's disease: a neurological disease of the brain causing progressive loss of memory and connectedness with societal expectations

Dementia: a neurological disease of the brain causing dissociated cognition and extensive confusion about the realities of life

Despair: complete and abject rejection of life as lived currently or in the past, without hope of anything positive to look forward to in the future

Ego transcendence: the psychosocial ability to minimize focus on self and to value and appreciate life and circumstances and other individuals that make life meaningful

Integrity: the psychosocial task for the elderly, according to Erikson, that is characterized by accepting and joyfully embracing the past, the present, and the future

Medicare: health care insurance for the elderly in the United States who have contributed to this fund during their working years and for those with severe disability and/or end stage renal disease. Medicare has three types of coverage: A for hospitalization, B for outpatient physician and diagnostic services, and D for prescription medications

Polypharmacy: a condition of being required to take multiple medications for multiple medical problems without professional oversight and selectivity regarding adverse reactions and/or drug-drug interactions

---

Physical and Physiological Characteristics

Elders, age 65 +, are the fastest growing population not only in the United States but in the entire world. Never in history has there been such a large number of people in this age group. This is mostly related to modern medical advances and interventions that allow these individuals to live longer. If healthy and active and fully cognitive, this is a true blessing. But when, on the other hand, elders are living with multiple medical problems, physical limitations, and pain, it becomes highly questionable that this could be considered a quality of life. A Healthy People 2020 priority objective is to attain high-quality longer lives free of preventable disease, disability, injury and premature death.

As discussed in the chapter on the Middle-aged adult, the human body after age 30 starts to decline. This decline continues in a definite downhill spiral in the elder years. This means that the immune system is compromised and there is increased risk for infection (especially respiratory infections like influenza and pneumonia) and an increased risk for cancer. Related to the decline in vision, hearing, mobility and balance, there is also an increased risk for falls and injuries. The body parts are simply wearing out.

Safety Concerns

Related to a decreased sense of balance and decreased visual acuity, it is essential that living quarters be made safe for the elder. This means that furniture should be arranged for ease of access and mobility. More open spacing, removal of throw rugs, and the installation of safety bars in tubs and showers are simple, yet effective ways to minimize the risk for falls. Some elders may also need to use a cane or walker to help them maintain stability when moving about.

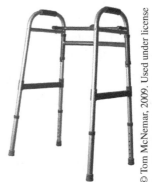

© Tom McNemar, 2009. Used under license from Shutterstock, Inc.

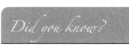
Did you know?

Have you ever had to depend on another to take you somewhere? Maybe your car was being repaired or you were too ill to drive yourself? An occasional event like this, for most of us, would be tolerable, but most individuals do not like to be in this dependent role on a routine basis. This is what elders face when they finally give up their driving privileges.

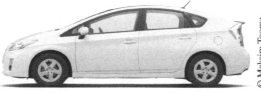

© Maksim Toome, 2011. Used under license from Shutterstock, Inc.

Driving is a major concern for the elderly. The slower response time and reduced visual acuity, especially in the peripheral vision, make driving a very risky endeavor. Even though safety is emphasized, most elders are reluctant to give up the car keys because that means giving up a major exercise of independence and freedom.

Related to lower metabolism and loss of subcutaneous tissue, most elderly individuals experience difficulty in temperature regulation. For the most part, the elderly tend to get cold or hot very easily. Oftentimes adjusting the thermostat to accommodate the preferences of the elderly could make it extremely uncomfortable for others in the same room.

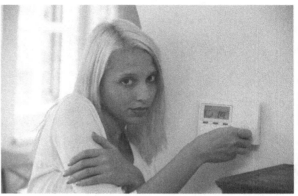

© Gina Sanders, 2009. Used under license from Shutterstock, Inc.

Also related to the loss of subcutaneous tissue, the skin of the elderly is extremely fragile. Without moisturizing lotions and protective padding of bony surfaces, the skin is extremely vulnerable to break down. Decubitus ulcers can and should be prevented.

Related to lower metabolism and generally speaking, minimal physical activity, the caloric intake for the elderly should be substantially less than in earlier years. There still is a great need for balanced nutrition (with some increased emphasis on fiber) and optimal hydration. Fiber and fluids are needed to help move ingested foods through the digestive track. It is not uncommon for many elders to be concerned about their bowel movements and most stay worried about constipation. The normal reduction in body fluids related to aging, and the fact that most elders are taking multiple medications, makes it necessary to drink at least 64 ounces of fluid per day. Unfortunately, most drink less than half this amount so then constipation does become a problem.

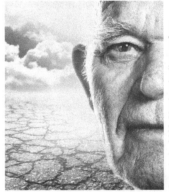

© Andrejs, 2009. Used under license from Shutterstock, Inc.

The low metabolism and relative inactivity of the elderly also makes them tend to sleep a lot. Actually, because of the inactivity, they need less sleep (5 to 6 hours of sleep per night), but most get 10 to 12 hours of sleep. Many elders nap frequently during the day making them restless through the night. For most elders, it is recommended that they be encouraged to stay awake and alert during the day so they can obtain an extended, restful sleep during the night.

Health Care Issues

Health care for the older adult is a major concern. The elder population is the greatest consumer of health care services and there are greater costs associated with elder health than for any other age group. Because elders are living longer, they are increasingly vulnerable to disease and suffer from multiple diseases or conditions that demand medical attention. Cancer occurs more readily in elders because the immune system becomes worn out with increased age, making mutations more likely to take place. And Dementia occurs more readily in elders because the neurons in the brain are less pliable and become entangled resulting in confusion and disorientation.

Adults over the age of 65 are eligible to receive Medicare part A if they have contributed to Social Security during their working years. Medicare part A only covers hospitalization so most older adults opt to have part B and part D as well. Part B covers doctor office visits and laboratory tests and part D covers prescription

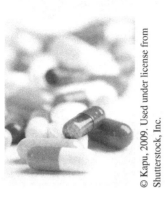

© Kapu, 2009. Used under license from Shutterstock, Inc.

medications. Under the Patient Protection and Affordable Care Act of 2010, Medicare now encourages older adults to stay well and get annual check-ups and screenings at little or no cost.

Because of modern pharmacotherapeutics and surgical interventions, life can be sustained for years well beyond what was possible in the past. Unfortunately, for most elder individuals, this means that they need to take many medications. **Polypharmacy** is a major concern for the elderly. Polypharmacy is a phenomenon that results from taking multiple prescription medications prescribed by multiple providers without coordinated oversight regarding possible adverse effects or drug-drug interactions.

When elders seek services from multiple providers for their multiple conditions (e.g., a cardiologist for coronary problems, a rheumatologist for arthritic dysfunctions, a gastroenterologist for digestive issues, an ophthamologist for vision problems), there is usually minimal communication between these specialists. The result is that there may be some medications prescribed for one condition that could counteract the effect of a medication prescribed for another condition, or the medications may actually potentiate or aggravate one of the other conditions.

This becomes an even bigger problem when prescriptions are filled at multiple pharmacies. When a single pharmacy is accessed, there is a greater likelihood that drug-drug interactions and adverse effects will be more readily identified.

A major contributor to polypharmacy is the fact that, in the health care delivery system today, specialists are sought by consumers without consultation with family physicians. This is especially true for the older adult. It would be much better, especially for the older adult, to have a primary care provider as a coordinator of care. This physician essentially would serve as the gatekeeper for the total care of the individual and would be the best hope to guard against polypharmacy.

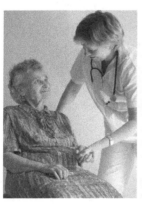

© Alexander Raths, 2009. Used under license from Shutterstock, Inc.

It is not uncommon at all for elders to have multiple chronic diseases like hypertension, diabetes, congestive heart failure, arthritis, and peripheral vascular disease. The pain and/or limitations associated with these conditions put major restrictions on the elder related to mobility and **activities of daily living**. Many elders require assistance to even get out of bed, to open their pill bottles, to prepare or cut food so it is edible, to dress and to bathe, and maybe even to get from point A to point B. It is not that family members or health care professionals do not like to assist in these activities, but it is a costly, time–consuming, and demanding task that causes caregiver burnout and the potential for elder abuse. From the elder perspective, this is a common cause of depression. Very few people like to have someone else take care of these very private and previously independent functions. It is humiliating and depressing. It is no wonder that so many elders experience depression.

Just as in middle age, the older adults generally desire to be respected for their accomplishments and they thrive on sharing their experiences and expertise. Most elders are very proud in their reminiscing and they need to share this to validate the meaningfulness of their life. Caregivers are highly encouraged to provide opportunities for this. Elders also need to have meaningful discussions about current events. Watching the news on TV, reading the newspaper, and reading books or journals keeps the elder mind active and helps elders to compare and contrast what is happening today against what they may have experienced in the past. The way things were is not necessarily passé—and it is fascinating to hear about what people went through to get us where we are today. There is a lot to be learned from elders and a lot to be grateful to them for.

Keeping the mind active is essential for elders. Reading, working crossword puzzles, playing bingo, and even playing cards helps the elder to stay cognitively alert. Experiencing momentary lapses in memory, commonly referred to as having a "senior moment," is very normal. There is a normal age-related physiological slowing in mental processing that requires a little longer time to remember names, numbers, or facts. But this decline in **fluid intelligence** is readily overshadowed by the flourishing of **crystallized intelligence**, that is, the wisdom that they have acquired through knowledge and life's experiences.

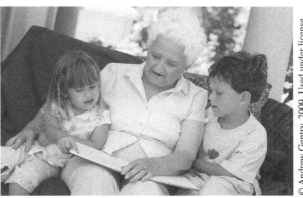

© Andrew Gentry, 2009. Used under license from Shutterstock, Inc.

Memory Loss

It is not uncommon at all for elders to have lapses in short term memory. They frequently cannot recall what they ate for dinner last evening or wore to Church the day before. But long term memory is usually quite intact. That is why elders are so eager to share stories of the 'good ole days'.

When there is extensive memory loss or confusion and an inability to remember how to perform normal activities of daily living, this most likely is dementia. **Dementia** is not normal in the elderly; it is a disease. The increasing number of elders with **Alzheimer's Disease**, a form of dementia, makes it seem like an inevitable occurrence, but this is completely false. Alzheimer's is a progressive deterioration of cognition resulting in complete dissociation with normal societal expectations. Even though the specific causes of Alzheimer's have not yet been identified, there are medications that may slow the process. Nonetheless, most individuals with Alzheimer's need to be cared for in a very tightly secured and safe environmental setting.

Dementia can occur at any age from brain injury or cerebral vascular accident, but is most often seen in elders as Alzheimer's disease. Alzheimer's disease is a type of dementia and is the most common type of dementia, accounting for up to 80% of cases and is most common seen in elders. Because Alzheimer's is characterized by plaques and tangles and inflammation in the brain cells which are only detectable post mortem, this disease is diagnosed by symptoms.

The characteristic symptoms of Alzheimer's are: memory loss, difficulty in problem solving for basic needs, confusion with time and place, difficulty understanding contrasting images and spatial relationships, gaps in speaking (struggling to find the words to complete the sentence), consistently losing or misplacing things and inability to retrace steps to recover, decreased judgment especially related to personal grooming and money matters, withdrawal from social gatherings and changes in mood and personality. (Alzheimer's .org 2015).

Alzheimer's disease is progressive in three distinct stages over a span of 4–20 years but there is no predictive pattern related to the amount of time that individuals will spend in each stage. In the early stage, short term memory lapses and difficulty in concentration, organization and planning are apparent, but individuals in this stage are usually able to continue to function independently. Caregivers are tasked with assisting these individuals with appointments and medications by using calendars, reminders and the establishment of a regular routine. Most Alzheimer patients in this initial stage may also need assistance with money management.

Because individuals realize that they forget things and misplace things, they sometime become agitated and frustrated. Family and caregivers should be aware of this and offer emotional support and encouragement and/or facilitate them in finding a support group.

In the second stage (usually the longest stage), individuals demonstrate an decreased ability to remember events in their own life and personal information such as where they lived previously, phone number and address, increased confusion about time and day of the week, withdrawal from social interaction and challenging situations, increased wandering, decreased ability in activities of daily living especially in bathing, dressing, grooming, and toileting, increased tendency to be combative (refusing to do things as requested), and changes in personality. Caregivers are tasked with 24 hour daily monitoring. Because this is an overwhelming task, caregivers need to have respite assistance and also need to make sure they are taking care of themselves. Because this is such a continuous strain, family members in caregiver roles, often find that placement in an Assisted Living facility or Nursing Home is a much more viable alternative.

In the final stage of Alzheimer's disease, individuals no longer respond to their surroundings and lose the ability to recognize familiar faces, communicate meaningfully, and often lose control of basic body functions such as eating, walking and toileting. These individuals usually require around the clock nursing care because they are so totally dependent on others for their basic needs and because they are increasingly prone to infection especially pneumonia. (Alzheimer's.org 2015)

Need for Companionship

Even if it is bingo or a quilting session, elders have a great need for companionship with people of their own age. Socialization is very important. These sessions provide opportunities for support and understanding and reminiscing.

B	I	N	G	O
6	24	37	49	66
12	21	39	46	73
15	22	FREE	48	74
14	23	36	47	75
13	19	44	55	72

© Scott Rothstein, 2009. Used under license from Shutterstock, Inc.

Need for Independence

Elders need to be independent and stay active as long as possible. Being able to walk and/or to drive means they can go and do what they want when they want. Once mobility is restricted, independence is severely compromised. Encouraging elders to participate in some form of exercise is critically important. Even if they are unable to walk briskly, they can at least take a relaxing stroll. Many elders are able to swim or do water aerobics and others can do chair exercises that stretch and tone their upper bodies. Others remain quite active with golf or tennis or gardening.

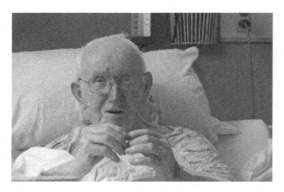
© Andrew Gentry, 2009. Used under license from Shutterstock, Inc.

Need for Assistance

Most elders do not like to ask for help but there are some who demand and expect help from their children and others. When this occurs, there is a high risk for elder abuse. **Elder abuse** may occur because the care-giving expectations are too demanding or stressful. The elder demands may interfere with routine family functions such as meals, outings, and/or vacations or with the need for personal time. In some families, caregivers have had to quit their jobs to take care of the elder. This may cause the caregiver to become resentful and may also place a significant financial burden on the family. To guard against this potential for burnout, caregivers are advised to seek alternative strategies. In most communities there are Adult Day Care centers where the elder individual can be cared for in a protected environment, while the caregiver maintains their working schedule and the family can function in a more normal routine. Assisted living facilities are also available for elders who need help with activities of daily living. Even though some of these facilities are available through Medicaid, most require a substantial fee that is not covered by Medicare or other insurance plans. There are long-term care insurance policies that cover these expenses, but the premiums are expensive and the policy must be held for a considerable amount of time before claims can be submitted.

Elder Abuse

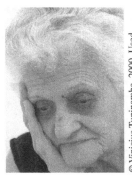

© Vinicius Tupinamba, 2009. Used under license from Shutterstock, Inc.

Elder abuse may take the form of isolation, verbal abuse, financial abuse, or physical abuse. For example, elders may be confined to their room until it is convenient for the caregiver to respond to their wants or needs. Elders may be put into diapers so that the caregiver is not bothered with assisting them to the restroom. Many elders are verbally abused and talked to like they are a child or even worse as an animal that is to do what they are told without any regard for what they may want. Some elders have their life savings literally wiped out by so-called caring helpers. And some elders are even subjected to hitting, pinching, pulling hair, and even sexual abuse, just because they asked for assistance.

Other elders, because they do not want to be a burden on others, don't ask for help when they need it. This also is not a good situation. They attempt to do things beyond their ability, resulting in preventable falls and fractures. They may also overfill the washing machine or dishwasher, resulting in preventable repairs and clean-up or leave the stove on resulting in fire. Elders may also not discuss medically apparent symptoms that are indicative of serious problems. The delay in seeking help then makes the condition even more serious or leads to complications that require extensive and prolonged treatment.

Developmental Theories

Integrity vs. Despair (Erikson)

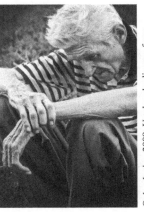

© dundanim, 2009. Used under license from Shutterstock, Inc.

According to Erikson (1969), the psychosocial task for elders is Integrity. **Integrity** is characterized by the ability to accept and embrace the past, the present, and the future. This is often referred to as **ego transcendence**, meaning that they are able to minimize focus on themselves and can appreciate the life they have and the other individuals that make that life meaningful.

Integrity means that the elderly need to look back on their lives and accept the good and bad without regret or resentment, that is, to come to terms with the fact that no matter what they did or didn't do, that they did the best they could under the circumstances. This is also a valid reason for allowing and encouraging the elderly to reminisce so they can put it all into perspective. Integrity also requires that the elderly accept their current status, whether this is health or a crippled broken body with extensive limitations. Body image is just as important to the elderly as it was during the teen years. They need to recognize that they will never be the same beautiful and intact individual that they once were and be okay with the normal aging processes that have become apparent and with any diseases that they may have acquired. This is very difficult for some and they become preoccupied with their physique and physical conditions. These elders focus on what is wrong rather than try to take joy in the capabilities that they do have. Integrity also means that the elderly need to come to terms with the fact that they will not live forever and that death is more imminent now than it has ever been. Accepting this fact helps them to put their lives in order so they will be able to die peacefully. It is not uncommon for many elderly to take an increased interest in spirituality to help them in this transition.

If integrity is not accomplished, despair becomes evident. **Despair** is the abject rejection of anything that life has to offer. Elders in despair exhibit the classic signs of depression (sadness, refusal to eat, increased sleep, poor posture) and tend to isolate themselves from social interaction. When encouraged to participate in activities, elders in despair persist in grumbling and groaning.

Depression can be treated with medication but, when elders truly experience despair, it is a very sad scenario that essentially cannot be overcome. Caregivers need to be alert to signs of despair in order to intervene early enough to try to help the elder to gain a more positive perspective. If despair persists, suicide is always a risk, but elders may die of "failure to thrive," even when there are no obvious physical causes.

Elders need to be respected and valued in our society. Whether they are healthy or ill, it is important to recognize their past contributions and their current place of value in our world. Even though health care has provided longevity to elders, there is an even greater need to meet the total holistic needs of the elderly. There is a major outcry for quality of life.

Cognition: Crystallized Intelligence/Wisdom (Piaget)

Elderly individuals who do not suffer from Alzheimer's Disease or dementia are wonderful historians and great communicators. They can recount events with delightful detail and can share a perspective only possible from someone who has experienced life to the fullest. This is "Wisdom" that comes from knowledge, experience and crystallized intelligence.

Morality: Universal Ethical Principles (Kohlberg)

As in middle age, the older adult is capable of doing the right thing for the right reason, because it is the right (ethical) thing to do. This is the stage of Universal Ethical Principles. But as discussed, just because they have this capability, does not mean that they always or consistently act in this manner. There may be times when they revert to lower levels of morality.

Summary

More and more people are growing old and living longer than ever before. If the older adult is healthy and active, this is a wonderful time of life. But because of the increased risk for disease and injury, polypharmacy and dementia, this is often a precarious time of life.

References

Alz.org. Dementia vs Alzheimers. Retrieved from www.alz.org on 5/25/2015.

Erikson, E. H. (1968). *Childhood and society* (35th anniversary ed.). New York: Norton.

Healthy People 2020 Framework (retrieved 12/17/2017 from www.healthypeople.gov).

Kohlberg, L. (1969). *The philosophy of moral development: Vol. 1*. San Francisco: Harper & Row.

Maslow, A. (1968). *Toward a psychology of being* (2nd ed.). New York: Van Nostrand-Reinhold.

Piaget, J. (1950). *The psychology of intelligence*. London: Routledge and Kegan Paul.

Reflection

In the space below, think of someone you know in this age group and describe something specific that they say or do that validates the theory as explained in this chapter

Assignment

Complete this form with essential data for the Older Adult

Growth and Development Guide for the Older Adult

	Physical Traits	Physical Abilities	Psychosocial Task (Erikson)	Evidence of How Achieved	Evidence of Non-Achievement	Cognitive Ability (Piaget)	Evidence of Achievement	Moral Capability (Kohlberg)	Evidence of Achievement
Older Adult (65+ years)									

Study Guide for
The Older Adult (65+ Years)

1/2. Relate the physiologic changes occurring in the older adult to their nutritional, sleep, elimination and thermal regulation needs.

3/4. Identify at least 2 physiologic changes that occur in the older adult that may impact activities of daily living and/or safety issues.

5. Describe how and why polypharmacy occurs in the older adult.

6. Describe how and why elder abuse occurs and identify at least 2 viable ways to prevent this from occurring.

7. Explain how integrity is achieved by the older adult.

8. Explain why elders may experience despair and/or depression.

9. Relate the cognitive ability of the older adult to recalling the past and the present.

10. Explain the difference between declining fluid intelligence and dementia.

Name: _____

Review

1. Which of the following statements by a 92-year-old man best describes achievement of Erikson's "Ego integrity"?
   a. "I have a lot of things wrong with me but I know that comes with the territory."
   b. "I have made many mistakes along the way and wish I had the chance to relive many years of my life."
   c. "I don't like being old and I don't like other people treating me like I am."
   d. "I don't like being old; I want to be young again and do all the things I did before."

2. Ego transcendence in the elderly is best described as…
   a. being disinterested in sustaining a sense of personal ego.
   b. being able to see through the egotistical comments of others.
   c. being aware of self in a realistic perspective.
   d. being superior to other generations in ego capabilities.

3. Which of the following is the greatest contributing factor to wrinkles in the older adult?
   a. loss of subcutaneous fat
   b. lack of hygiene
   c. failure to apply moisturizer
   d. decrease in vitamin A

4. Why are older adults at higher risk to have cancer?
   a. age-related loss of fluid in the body
   b. decline in immune response
   c. poor nutrition
   d. lack of exercise

G&D: The Older Adult

- Fastest growing segment of population
  - Medical advances
  - Healthier environments
- Healthy People 2020 Goal
  - To Increase Years of Healthy Living
    - Longevity without quality of life is not desirable
      - Disease / Pain / Immobility

© Andrew Gentry, 2009

Images used under license from Shutterstock, Inc.

Live longer w/ higher quality of life

G&D: The Older Adult

- Physiologic Appearance
  - Loss in height
  - Wrinkles
  - Gray hair
- Physiologic Changes
  - Loss of subcutaneous fat
    - Loss of thermal insulation
    - Increased risk for skin breakdown
  - Loss of fluid
    - Loss of balance / kinesthetic sense

© Andrejs Pidjass, 2009

© Alexander Raths, 2009

Images used under license from Shutterstock, Inc.

*Skin becomes delecate have to change position to prevent ulcers (pressure)

G&D: The Older Adult

- Physiologic Decline
  - Immune response
    - Increased risk for respiratory infections
    - Increased risk for cancer
  - Sensory perception
    - Deficits in vision, hearing, taste
      - Glasses
      - Hearing aids
      - ??? Ability to safely drive a car
  - Flexibility
    - Increased risk for falls
    - May need ambulation assistive devices

© Maksim Toome, 2011

© digitallife, 2009.

Images used under license from Shutterstock, Inc.

G&D: The Older Adult

- Slower Metabolism in Elders
  - Fewer calories needed
    - Need balanced nutrition
  - Less sleep but most sleep more
  - Exercise essential for circulation
    - Arm chair exercises if mobility limited
  - Problems with Constipation
    - Need fiber
  - Longer time for medication absorption

Need

Constipation due to dehydration, lack of fiber.

G&D: The Older Adult

- Health Care Concerns
  - Medicare Wellness Challenge
  - Medicare Costs
  - Multiple chronic conditions
    - Diabetes
    - Arthritis
    - Hypertension
  - Multiple health care providers
    - Specialists vs. Generalists
    - Gerontologists vs. Specialists
  - Multiple medications
    - Polypharmacy
    - Medications to counter effects of other medicines

© Mirek Kijewski, 2011

Images used under license from Shutterstock, Inc.

Medicare = age 65 - A - Hospital
B = 80% only covered - Dr. office visits / labs
D = medication / drugs

Polypharmacy - multiple Meds.

G & D: The Older Adult

- Elder Limitations
  - Activities of Daily Living
    - Eating
      - Eye-hand coordination
      - Teeth
    - Dressing
      - Buttons / snaps
    - Bathing
      - Getting in and out of tub/shower
      - Bending to wash and/or dry
    - Toileting
      - Timing
      - Cleansing
    - Ambulation
      - Stability
      - Mobility

© Alexander Raths, 2009

© digitalife, 2009

Images used under license from Shutterstock, Inc.

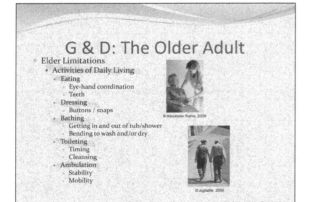

High rate of mortality if fall

Ambulate = open spacing - making environment safe

G & D: The Older Adult

Senility means "OLD"; not forgetful
- Some short term memory loss associated with loss of fluid intelligence
  - Takes longer to make the neural connections
- Long term memory intact
- Disorientation is not normal even though
- Alzheimer's IS more common among elderly

© argus, 2009

Images used under license from Shutterstock, Inc.

think if there is medication affecting.
Alzheimers Not cureable

G&D: The Older Adult

- Memory Loss
  - Intermittent short term memory lapse
  - Dementia
  - Alzheimers

G&D: The Older Adult

- Need for
  - Companionship
  - Independence
  - Assistance

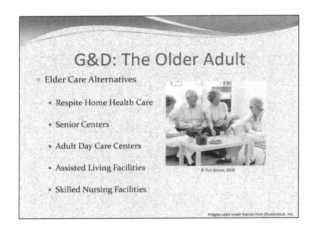

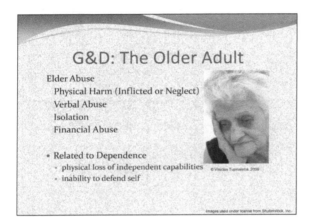

G&D: The Older Adult

- INTEGRITY (Erikson)
  - Realistic perspective of
    - Past: accept without regret
      - Love to reminisce
      - Can laugh about mistakes
    - Present: Body image; limitations
    - Future: death
  - Ego Transcendence

- DESPAIR
  - Regret
  - Body Preoccupation
  - Unhappiness

Integrity = acceptance.
Ego transcendence = positive/realistic
view on life.

G&D: The Older Adult

- Cognition (Piaget)
  - Crystallized Intelligence
    - Elders deserve respect
    - Years of experience and Wisdom
    - Have a lot to share

- Fluid Intelligence
  - Sustained through keeping up with current events
  - Crossword puzzles / Bingo / Cards

Fluid Intelligence — keeping mind active, Physical Activity

G&D: The Older Adult

- Morality (Kohlberg)
  - Universal Ethical Principles
    - Doing the right thing for the right reason
    - Because it is the right (ethical) thing to do

Doing

Family Health

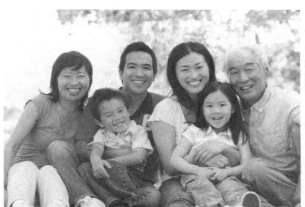

© Monkey Business Images, 2009. Used under license from Shutterstock, Inc.

Objectives

Upon completion of this chapter, the reader should be able to:

1. Define and describe family in terms of structure and function.
2. Differentiate the different types of families and describe roles and functions typically assumed by family members.
3. Construct a genogram and ecomap as a means of family assessment.
4. Compare and contrast Systems, Developmental, and Structure/Function models of family assessment.
5. Describe family tasks as described by Duvall and Miller and relate these tasks to the individual life stages tasks as described by Erikson.
6. Identify common concerns and challenges experienced by families during the various stages of development.

Key Terms

EcoMap: an assessment tool that evaluates the strength of social interpersonal interactions

Family: an alliance of interacting individuals who are related by blood, marriage, cohabitation, or adoption and who are interdependent in carrying out relevant functions through roles

Family Developmental Stages: a schema of challenges (tasks) for families, developed by Duvall and Miller, and based on progressive stages of development; an adaptation of Erikson's Psychosocial theory to a family perspective

Functional Health Patterns: patterns (routines) of behavior, identified by Gordon, that define health/non-health of families and individuals

Genogram: an assessment tool that tracks biologic and disease predispositions in families based on a three generational analysis

Hierarchy of Needs: an ascending perspective, as described by Maslow, of how individuals and families aspire and achieve their optimal potentials

Launching: the process by which parents prepare and successfully release their young adult children into society to be independent, self–reliant, and maturely functioning adults.

Structure/Function Assessment: an assessment tool that describes family types and their dependent and independent functioning patterns.

Systems Theory: a strategic assessment instrument that is characterized by structural boundaries and the on-going interchange of energy between boundaries

Definition of Family

No discussion about Growth and Development is complete without an analysis of family. Individuals grow and develop within families and it is through the interaction of family members that most developmental tasks are achieved. Families may be biological or sociological or both in origin. In the following paragraphs, different types of families will be described as well as family roles and responsibilities.

Family, by definition, is an alliance of interacting individuals who are related by blood, marriage, cohabitation, or adoption and who are interdependent in carrying out relevant functions through roles. By this definition, it is obvious that members of communes, members of foster homes, same sex unions/marriages, and cohabiting individuals are all considered to be family members. It is the assumption of roles and the interdependence that are the major commonalities.

Family Assessment

Structure/Function Model

There are multiple models that can be used for assessing families. One of these models, the **Structure/Function Assessment** model, is simply descriptive. Structure defines the size and type of the family and who the family members are (age, sex) and Function defines the roles assumed by the family members.

There are many family structural types. A person may be single, self-supporting, and living alone and still be a member of a family because they have an extended family or social support system that still allows them to function in an identified role and in an interdependent manner. The traditional family (Mom, Dad, children) is also known as a nuclear family. When family homes become residences for other transgenerational family members (grandparents, sisters, brothers, nieces, nephews, and cousins), or even close friends, the family is described as an extended family. When divorced individuals with children remarry, this is known as a blended or merged family. There is a double blending when the spouse also is divorced with children. There are also many single-parent families, either by choice, death, or divorce, in which the parent assumes roles otherwise shared with a partner. Cohabitating families include homosexual unions (now legal marriages), members of communes, and rent-sharing heterosexuals.

Function describes the role(s) that each member assumes. These roles address familiar household responsibilities such as being the provider (bread winner) or the stay at home manager, the bill payer, the child care overseer for everyday goals and discipline (when children are part of the picture), or the decision maker over issues affecting the entire family. Roles are also assumed for ordinary everyday chores such as cleaning the house, cooking, transporting, yard work, and garbage patrol. Some informal roles assumed by family members include being the nurturer (the calming, soother), the problem solver (the one with insight to anticipate and solve problems), the peacemaker (the one who intervenes to minimize negative and argumentative discussions), the organizer (the one who is always planning trips, outings, games, etc.), the nay-sayer (the one who never wants to do what everyone else wants to do), the passive complier (the one who never has an opinion about family choices—just goes along for the ride), the devil's advocate (the one who always presents an alternative just to keep everyone open to alternative possibilities), and the scapegoat (the one who always get blamed when things go wrong). While this list is not all-inclusive, it is representative of roles assumed by many families.

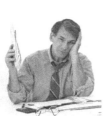
© forestpath, 2009. Used under license from Shutterstock, Inc.

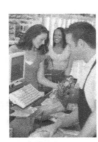
© Monkey Business Images, 2009. Used under license from Shutterstock, Inc.

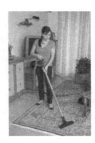
© Gina Sanders, 2009. Used under license from Shutterstock, Inc.

The Structure/Function model also addresses roles that are assumed outside of the home whether it is work related or with an emphasis on personal satisfaction. This could include volunteer interests as well as sports or music participation and/or enjoyment.

The Structure/Function model is also used to assess values, interaction patterns, and coping. Values include cultural and religious orientations, use of leisure time, and perspectives on education and health. Some families routinely do many things together (sharing family meals, attending church services, going on vacation), while other families may thrive on individual pursuit of excellence or satisfaction.

Did you know?

Do you think that families are healthier and happier if they go and do things together? This may well be true if the family members value these activities. But what if the family members resent these activities? On the other hand, there may be families who may not have the opportunity or time to coordinate family activities but feel the love and support of their family members. These families may feel more loyal and happy than families that are constantly on the unified go.

Interaction patterns include ways of expressing affection, love, sorrow, and anger. Some families are very warm and fuzzy and engage in frequent hugs and kisses, while other families are far more reserved in these outward signs of affection and yet are extremely supportive of one another and are always available and willing to help where and when needed. Another interaction pattern that is critical to family functioning is the extent of openness of communication between family members.

Some families are very spontaneous in sharing feelings and thoughts about what they are doing, while others tend to have these discussions only if and when there is a concern. Interaction patterns are simply evidence of awareness of the significance of family members in each individual's life. There really is no right or wrong; it is good if it works for the family and the individual members within that family.

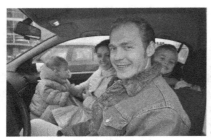
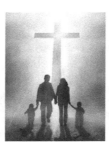
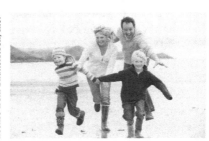

Coping is essentially a response to adversity. Coping addresses the degree of emotional support that is offered to the other family members, the availability of support outside the immediate family circle, identification of common sources of stress, common methods of handling stressful situations and conflicting goals of family members, and the financial ability to meet current needs as well as wants.

Using the Structure/Function model, family strengths and weaknesses can readily be identified. Healthy families tend to have strong personal, social, and spiritual values. They are respectful of one another and flexible in adapting to change. They are strongly loyal to and supportive of one another. These healthy families also have open meaningful communication and evidence healthy child-rearing practices. One of the greatest assets of healthy families is their willingness to offer help when and where needed but they are also willing to accept and receive help when they need it.

Helpful Tools for Assessing Families Using the Structure/Function Model

There are two assessment tools that are especially helpful when assessing families using the Structure Function Model. The first is a **Genogram**. A genogram is a three-generational analysis of family structure and changes resulting from births, adoptions, marriage/re-marriage, and death. A genogram can also be used to identify character traits or tendencies such as "heavy drinker" or "chain smoker" or "has anger management issues." And genograms are applicable to same sex unions/marriages as well as for traditional nuclear families. On this schematic, family member ages, occupations, behavioral lifestyles and diseases can readily be added. A **genogram** is often used to quickly identify biological risks and family predispositions to disease or dysfunction. Biological and/or genetic factors are predispositions that usually cannot be altered, but families can at least be aware of risks and seek medical attention in a timely manner. See example below.

Genogram: Structure/Risk factors

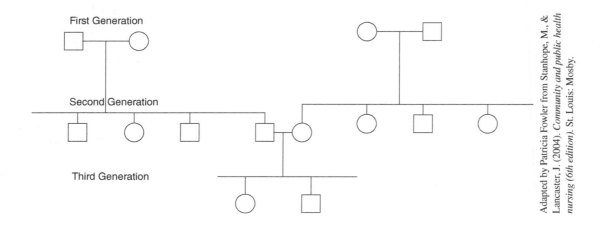

Adapted by Patricia Fowler from Stanhope, M., & Lancaster, J. (2004). *Community and public health nursing (6th edition)*. St. Louis: Mosby.

A genogram is an effective tool to aid the health care provider in recognizing familial traits that put family members at increased risk for certain diseases. But it is up to the family to choose to adapt to healthy lifestyle behaviors and/or obtain the precautionary screenings that might be indicated.

The second assessment tool is the **Ecomap**. This too is a quick pictorial of interactions between the family members and their outside contacts. The width of the arrows indicates the strength of the relationships and the direction of the arrows indicates the source and destination of the feeling about the relationship. See example below. In same sex unions/marriages, the ecomap recognizes two spouses as opposed to the nuclear family husband/wife model depicted below.

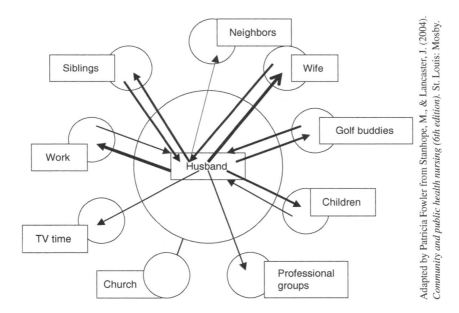

Adapted by Patricia Fowler from Stanhope, M., & Lancaster, J. (2004). *Community and public health nursing (6th edition).* St. Louis: Mosby.

Systems Model

As true as it is that individuals cannot be assessed without factoring in the influences of the family, the same can be said regarding families. Families cannot be assessed without factoring in the environment in which they exist. The Systems Model, depicted below, shows that, even though family integrity and values establish a safe core boundary of structure and function, there is a constant interchange of energy between the multiple dimensions of existence outside the family.

Systems

Structural and functional boundaries/energy exchange

Do you think it is healthy for families to limit their outside involvement? Some families think that all available free time should be devoted to family activity but family members need to be able to express their individual interests in order to achieve their aspirations to self-actualization.

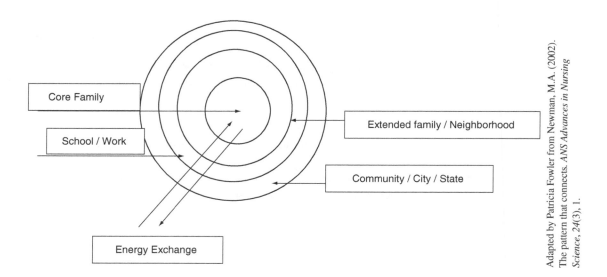

Adapted by Patricia Fowler from Newman, M.A. (2002). The pattern that connects. *ANS Advances in Nursing Science*, *24*(3), 1.

Functional Health Patterns

Gordon (1994) created an additional assessment framework that evaluates health lifestyle patterns for individuals and for families. The **functional health patterns** described by Gordon are holistic, that is, consider the multiple dimensions of health without exclusive focus on the biologic concerns. Gordon's functional health patterns include: Health Perception and Management, Nutrition, Elimination, Sleep/Rest, Cognitive and Perceptual ability, Self-Perception and Self-Concept, Roles and Relationships, Sexuality, Coping and Stress tolerance, and Values and Beliefs. Using Gordon's framework, it is readily seen that familiarity with foundational behaviors within the context of family (how we are brought up) is a strong predictor of individual future preferences.

Health perception and management includes an awareness of the existing health status of each family member as well as health promotion/preventive practices, and how and when they seek medical attention. Some families only seek medical care in life-threatening situations and others run to the doctor for every scraped knee. A healthy family recognizes the difference and responds from a balanced perspective. Relating to health care, many risks are linked with health insurance coverage. With insurance, families tend to seek health care; without health insurance they do not. This may become a renewed concern since the Tax Reform Bill (2017) removed the mandate for everyone to have health care insurance that was required under the Affordable Health Care Act (2010). There is also concern related to eligibility for spousal benefits (that includes health care insurance) which may or may not be granted in some states for same sex partners, unions/marriages. Availability of health care services is another concern. If there are no services offered after 5:00 P.M. or on the week-end, it can be well understood that families may seek health care services in the emergency room, even though this is inappropriate.

Illness and injury impact family function, no matter what type the family is or what their functions are. The extent of this impact is dependent upon the nature of the illness (whether it is minor or life threatening), the duration of the illness (2 days vs. 2 years), the residual effects of the illness (permanent disability that forever shifts roles), the significance of the illness to the family system, the strength of the family-coping processes (including the strength of their resources and support system), the financial impact of the illness (loss of income, insurance coverage), and the effect of the illness on future family functioning.

Family health is often defined by lifestyle, biological, and environmental factors. The environmental risks associated with air, noise, water, and soil pollution cannot always be corrected, but when families are aware of the negative impact, hopefully they will choose to remove themselves from the source. Lifestyle behaviors related to nutrition, sleep, stress management, and the effective use of leisure can be very positive but also very damaging to family integrity. Gordon (1994) identifies nutrition, elimination, and sleep/rest as essential to family health. Eating healthily or not, and sleeping on a routine schedule or not, are patterns that are established early within families and are closely linked with family values. Other values evident in family functioning include education. If this is a priority, reading and learning are expectations rather than occasional pastimes and success in school is encouraged and rewarded rather than tolerated.

Family Developmental Stages

An alternate means of assessing families is in the application of Duvall and Miller's (1985) **Family Developmental Stages**. This model of assessment obviously does not apply in families in which there are no children. Duvall and Miller, adapted Erikson's (1965) Psychosocial theory, with age-related developmental tasks, to a family perspective. Duvall and Miller categorized families into critical stages: Beginning Families (couple, child bearing), Families with Preschoolers, Families with School-aged children, Families with Adolescents, Family with Young Adults, Families with Middle-aged adults, and Families with Elder Adults.

In the Beginning Families stage, the cohabitating or newlywed couples are challenged with the tasks of combining, changing, or adapting the routines and values of two very different individuals from two very different child-rearing families into a newly formed, unique pattern of functioning. This can be as complicated as finances or as simple as how to do the laundry, but it definitely requires communication, negotiation, and adaptation.

Then, the couple is challenged with the possibility of children. Whether they choose to start a family or choose to minimize this possibility, there are additional concerns and adaptations that must be made. There are many issues that need to be resolved, such as to use or not to use contraception, to seek fertility counseling or to let nature take its course, to be willing to put one's career on hold or not, and to be willing to give up alcohol for the duration of a pregnancy or not. Then, if and when pregnancy does occur, there are new concerns about the health of the fetus and the possibility of pre-maturity or birth defects.

In homosexual marriages, the decision to have or not have children, has different concerns. The couples may choose to adopt a child. Or they may choose to have their own children. Male couples may want to contribute their own sperm and have a surrogate mother. Female couples may want one of them to become impregnated by donor sperm and then carry the baby to term.

Once the baby is born, there are added concerns about Sudden Infant Death Syndrome (SIDS) and the multiple possibilities for injury or illness to this tiny, vulnerable offspring. During the infant's first year of life, parents are focused on meeting the dependency needs of their child, that is, the parents are helping the infant to learn to trust that the parents will respond to their needs. During the toddler and pre-school years, parents are then challenged to help the child to establish a sense of autonomy and initiative and in the school-age years, to help the child learn how to be successful in industrious endeavors.

As is apparent, in this schema, the family tasks, especially in the early years, are essentially similar to the developmental task of the oldest child in the family, that is, are focused on helping the oldest child to achieve their expected developmental task. Because it is the first time that young parents are encountering the challenge of the particular growth and developmental stage of their oldest child, the family needs to learn new and different strategies and make adaptations to succeed in this challenge. For example, there may be siblings in the home of pre-school age or school age, but the parents have dealt with the growth and developmental needs of these stages previously. It is the challenge of the first adolescent that turns their life upside down. Even though each child in a family is unique, there are certain commonalities that help parents to cope more efficiently and less stressfully the second or third time around.

According to Duvall and Miller's Family with Young Adults stage, parents are challenged to **launch** these young adults into the world as independent, self-sufficient adults. In the Family with Middle-aged adults, families are challenged to peak in their careers, to re-establish their spousal relationship (after the children are gone) and to prepare for retirement. In the Family with Elder adults stage, individuals are challenged to accept and embrace life in the past as well as in the present, and to prepare for the inevitability of death.

Within families, as with individuals, there is a **hierarchy of needs** that follows Maslow's (1968) description. The biological needs of air, food, water, and shelter are far more essential than safety and security, love and belonging, self-esteem, and self-actualization.

Maslow's Hierarchy of Needs

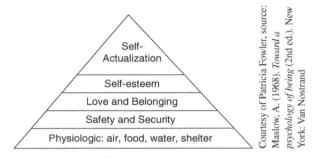

Courtesy of Patricia Fowler, source: Maslow, A. (1968). *Toward a psychology of being* (2nd ed.). New York: Van Nostrand

As described, there are multiple approaches and instruments available for assessing and/or describing families. They are all equally valid approaches but depending on the purpose, one or the other may work better in any given situation. An important thing to remember in Growth and Development, families and societies grow and develop as well as the individuals who make up these families and societies. So back to the beginning question, is it nature or nurture that makes us who we are? It definitely is BOTH!

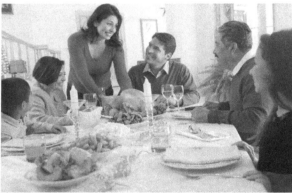

© Monkey Business Images, 2009. Used under license from Shutterstock, Inc.

Summary

Because no one lives in complete isolation of some familial influence, it is important for health care providers to understand this impact. In today's society, we now recognize multiple types of families. Each family is unique in its structure, function, interactions and risks. Family assessments help health care providers to recognize potential strengths and weaknesses and provide quality health care to the individuals in the family as well as to the family as a whole.

References

CNN Money: with contributions from Jeanne Sahadi, Kathryn Vasel, Tami Luhby, Anna Bahney, Jackie Wattles, Katie Lobosco, Lydia DePillis and Matt Egan. (Retrieved January 12, 2018 from http://money .cnn.com/2017/12/20/news/economy/republican-tax-reform-everything-you-need-to-know/index.html)

Duvall, E. M., & Miller, B. (1985). *Marriage and family development* (7th ed.). New York: Harper Collins.

Erikson, E. H. (1968). *Childhood and society* (35th anniversary ed.). New York: Norton.

Gordon, M. (1994). *Nursing diagnosis: Process and application* (3rd ed.). St. Louis: Mosby.

Kohlberg, L. (1969). *The philosophy of moral development: Vol. 1.* San Francisco: Harper & Row.

Maslow, A. (1968). *Toward a psychology of being* (2nd ed.). New York: Van Nostrand-Reinhold.

Newman, M. A. (2002). The pattern that connects. *ANS Advances in Nursing Science, 24*(3), 1.

Piaget, J. (1950). *The psychology of intelligence.* London: Routledge and Kegan Paul.

Stanhope, M., & Lancaster, J. (2004). *Community and public health nursing* (6th ed.). St. Louis: Mosby.

Reflection

In the space below, think about your own family and describe what you consider to be a strength or weakness as explained in this chapter.

Assignment

Construct a three generational genogram of your own family and identify ages, occupations, behavioral lifestyles of members (ex. smoker, drinks alcohol excessively, uses recreational drugs, exercises daily, etc.) as well as known disease and/or disease risks,

Name: _____

Study Guide for Family Health

1. Define Family.

2. Give examples of 3 different types of families and explain how each type fits the definition of family.

3. Differentiate structure from function as related to Family assessment.

4. Differentiate formal from informal family roles and give at least 2 examples of each.

5. Identify the 14 functional health patterns according to Gordon and explain how these can patterns relate to families as well as to individuals.

6. Explain how the developmental tasks for families with children relate to the developmental tasks of the individual family members.

7. Describe what a genogram is and how it is used in family assessment.

8. Describe what an ecomap is and how it is used in family assessment.

9. Describe Maslow's Hierarchy of Needs as it relates to family functioning.

10. Explain why family assessment is an important component is providing quality health care.

Name: _____

Review

1. Which is TRUE about the developmental tasks associated with Duval and Miller's Family Life Cycle Stage?

   a. They remain constant throughout the family's existence.
   b. They often clash with individual member's psychosocial needs.
   c. They change with the birth of each new child.
   d. They tend to correspond with meeting the tasks of the oldest child.

2. Which of the following is an effective instrument for assessing family sociologic risks? Choose all that apply.

   a. systems schema
   b. ecomap
   c. genogram
   d. Gordon's functional health patterns

3. Which family assessment tool evaluates health risks within three generations?

   a. Gordon's functional health patterns
   b. genogram
   c. ecomap
   d. system schema

4. What is the best descriptor of 'function' as it relates to family assessment?

   a. the birth order of family members
   b. the hidden talents of individual family members
   c. the occupation of each family member
   d. the role each family member has in family interdependence and relationships

G&D: FAMILY

- FAMILY Definition
  - an alliance of interacting individuals who are related by blood, marriage, cohabitation or adoption and who are interdependent in carrying out relevant functions through roles

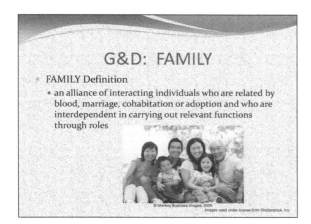

© Monkey Business Images, 2009
Images used under license from Shutterstock, Inc.

G&D: FAMILY

- FAMILY Types
  - Traditional (Nuclear)
    - Mom / Dad / Children
  - Non-traditional
    - Re-constituted: previous marriages with or without children
      - Blended or Merged families
    - Homosexual Unions (legal marriages)
    - Adoption
    - Extended family (transgenerational)
    - Cohabitating couples
    - Communes
    - Foster homes

G&D: FAMILY

- Describing Family by Structure
  - Size
  - Birth order
  - Age / sex of members
- Describing Family by Function
  - Roles
    - Breadwinner / bill payer
    - Daily activity (cooking, cleaning)
    - Childrearing (discipline)
    - Decision Maker
    - Nurturer
    - Peacemaker

© forestpath, 2009

© Gina Sanders, 2009
Images used under license from Shutterstock, Inc.

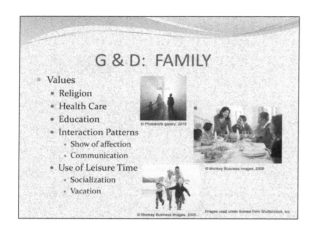

G & D: FAMILY

- Family Health Risk Assessment:
  - GENOGRAM
  - Can be used for same sex unions/marriages as well
  - Identifies family members and traits

Adapted by Patricia Fowler from Stanhope, M., & Lancaster, J. (2004). Community and public health nursing (6th edition). St. Louis. Mosby.

G & D: FAMILY

- Family Social Risk
  - ECOMAP (In same sex unions/marriages, there would be spouse/spouse rather than husband/wife)

Adapted by Patricia Fowler from Stanhope, M., & Lancaster, J. (2004). Community and public health nursing (6th edition). St. Louis. Mosby.

Genogram: for health risk assessment.

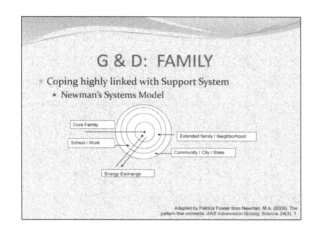

G & D: FAMILY

- Coping highly linked with Support System
  - Newman's Systems Model

Adapted by Patricia Fowler from Newman, M.A. (2002). The pattern that connects. *ANS Advances in Nursing Science*, 24(3), 1.

G&D: FAMILY

- Functional Health Patterns (Gordon)
  - Health Perception and Management,
  - Nutrition, Elimination,
  - Sleep/Rest,
  - Cognitive and Perceptual ability,
  - Self Perception and Self-Concept,
  - Roles and Relationships,
  - Sexuality,
  - Coping and Stress tolerance and
  - Values and beliefs.

© Monkey Business Images, 2009

Images used under license from Shutterstock, Inc.

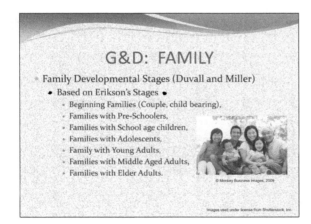

Based on the oldest child.

G&D: FAMILY

- Family Developmental Stages (Duvall and Miller)
  - Based on Erikson's Stages
    - Beginning Families (Couple, child bearing),
    - Families with Pre-Schoolers,
    - Families with School age children,
    - Families with Adolescents,
    - Family with Young Adults,
    - Families with Middle Aged Adults,
    - Families with Elder Adults.

© Monkey Business Images, 2009

Images used under license from Shutterstock, Inc.

G & D: FAMILY

Hierarchy of Needs (Maslow)

Self-Actualization
Self-esteem
Love and Belonging
Safety and Security
Physiologic: air, food, water, shelter

Courtesy of Patricia Fowler. source: Maslow, A. (1968). *Toward a psychology of being* (2nd ed.). New York: Van Nostrand

Index

A

Acne/perspiration, 121
Activities of daily living (ADL), 172
ADHD. *See* Attention Deficit Hyperactivity Disorder
ADL. *See* Activities of daily living
Adolescence (12–18 years)
  body image, 121–122
  developmental theories
    formal operations, 124–125
    identity vs. role diffusion, 123–124
    social system and development of conscience, 125
  emotional maturation, 122–123
  health concerns, 126
  health maintenance, 121
  hormone influence, 119–121
  parental challenges, 125–126
  and puberty
    physical growth spurt, 118–119
Alzheimer's disease, 173, 176
Amoral stage, for pregnancy, 37
Anticipatory guidance, developmental milestones for, 34
Apgar assessment, 27, 29
Asynchronous growth, 8
Attention Deficit Hyperactivity Disorder (ADHD), 100–101
Autonomy vs. shame and doubt
  emotion control, 57
  toilet training, 56–57

B

Benign prostatic hypertrophy (BPH) condition, 156
Blended/merged family, 190
Body dysmorphia, 122
Body system development, of infants, 32–33
Bonding, 30
BPH condition. *See* Benign prostatic hypertrophy condition
Bulimia, 122

C

Cause and effect, 80
Centering, 80
Cephalocaudal growth, 7
Childproofing, 55
Chronic illness, for middle age, 156
Classification, concrete operations stage, 100

Cognition theory (Jean Piaget)

concrete operations, for school age, 99–101
crystallized intelligence/wisdom
  middle age (35–65 years), 158
  older adult (65+ years), 176
formal operations
  adolescence (12–18 years), 124–125
  middle age (35–65 years), 158
  young adult (18–35 years), 141–142
pregnancy (first year of life), 36
preoperational and preconceptual thought,
  for toddler, 58
preoperational, for preschooler, 79–81
stages of, 9–11
Cohabitating families, 191
Common illnesses, of toddler, 59
Concrete operations stage, 10–11
  hobbies, 99–100
  learning, 100–101
  school, 100
Conservation of matter, 100
Conventional morality (Lawrence Kohlberg), 101
Conventional stage, growth and development, 13
Cooperative play, 75
Crystallized intelligence, 158, 173, 176

D

Dating, 120
Delayed gratification, 57
Dementia, 173
Depression, 124
Despair vs. integrity, 175–176
Development
  of conscience and social system, 125
  family stages, 195–196
  and growth
    nature vs. nurture, 5–8
    theory related to optimal nursing care, 4–8
  milestones, for anticipatory guidance, 34
  pre-natal considerations on fetal, 28–29
  principles of, 8
  theories, 15
    amoral stage, 37
    cognition theory, 9–11, 36